Writing Forensic Reports

Daniel P. Greenfield, MD, MPH, MS, is a practicing psychiatrist, addiction medicine specialist, and preventive medicine specialist. He was educated at Oberlin College, the University of North Carolina, the University of London, Rutgers University, and Harvard University. In addition to his clinical and forensic practice, Dr. Greenfield teaches at the Albert Einstein College of Medicine, where he is an attending physician at Montefiore Medical Center (Bronx, New York), and at Seton Hall University, where he is Clinical Professor of Neuroscience (Psychiatry) at the New Jersey Neuroscience Institute/JFK Medical Center (South Orange and Edison, New Jersey). Dr. Greenfield has lectured, published, and testified widely in areas of his background, training, and expertise, in academic, business, community, courtroom, government, and professional forums, as well as on television and radio.

Jack A. Gottschalk, JD, MA, MSM, is a best-selling author and a frequent television and radio guest. A lawyer and former prosecutor, he has appeared on *Court TV* and was the host of a cable TV show, *Legally Speaking.* In addition to writing and television appearances, Professor Gottschalk has appeared before community, business, and academic audiences, including the U.S. Naval War College and the Medill School of Journalism of Northwestern University.

He holds a law degree and graduate degrees in management and international relations and did additional graduate work at Columbia University. He is an adjunct faculty member at the Stillman School of Business of Seton Hall University.

Writing Forensic Reports

A Guide for Mental Health Professionals

Daniel P. Greenfield, MD, MPH, MS
Jack A. Gottschalk, JD, MA, MSM

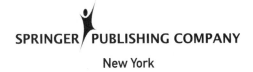

SPRINGER PUBLISHING COMPANY

New York

Springer Publishing Company, LLC
11 West 42nd Street
New York, NY 10036
www.springerpub.com

Acquisitions Editor: Sheri W. Sussman
Production Editor: Julia Rosen
Cover design: David Levy
Composition: Apex CoVantage, LLC

09 10 11 12/ 5 4 3 2 1

Library of Congress Cataloging-in-Publication Data

Greenfield, Daniel P.
Writing forensic reports : a guide for mental health professionals / Daniel P. Greenfield, Jack A. Gottschalk.
    p. ; cm.
Includes bibliographical references and index.
ISBN 978-0-8261-2158-5 (alk. paper)
1. Evidence, Expert. 2. Forensic psychiatry. 3. Medical writing. 4. Report writing.
I. Gottschalk, Jack A. II. Title.
[DNLM: 1. Forensic Psychiatry—methods. 2. Medical Records—legislation & jurisprudence. 3. Writing. W 740 G812w 2009]
RA1056.G64 2009
614'.1—dc22   2008038972

Printed in the United States of America by Bang Printing.

P

Daniel P. Greenfield, MD, MPH, MS, dedicates this book to his parents, who would have read and enjoyed it; to his wife and children and their families, who will probably read bits and pieces of the book and probably enjoy them; to his brother and sister-in-law and their children and families, who think the idea of the book is "neat"; and to Alma, his granddaughter, who is too young to read the book now, but who will certainly grow into it.

Jack A. Gottschalk, JD, MA, MSM, dedicates the book to Mom, Beverly, and Misty.

Contents

Foreword

In earlier times lawyers, juries, and judges could resolve criminal and civil issues cases, relying on their general knowledge and common sense both in preparing and in deciding a case. This is no longer so. As described in their work, *Writing Forensic Reports: A Guide for Mental Health Professionals,* Professors Daniel P. Greenfield and Jack Gottschalk address one discipline—psychiatry—in the vast array of disciplines in which forensic techniques are employed to assist legal practitioners and the courts.

The federal and state courts of the United States have established rules for the admission into evidence of otherwise inadmissible opinions of experts. Federal Evidence Rule 702 provides that if specialized knowledge "will assist the trier of fact to understand the evidence or to determine a fact in issue, a witness qualified as an expert by knowledge, skill, experience, training or education, may testify thereto in the form of opinion or otherwise."

The United States Supreme Court has mandated that federal trial courts exercise a gatekeeping function when determining the admissibility of proposed expert testimony under Rule 702, *Daubert v. Merrill Dow Pharm, Inc.,* 509 U.S. 579 (1993). The court must scrutinize with care the proposed expert testimony to ensure, first, that the expert is qualified, that is, that he is truly an expert in the field about which he proposes to report or testify; and second, that the process or techniques the expert used in formulating the opinion are reliable, that is, that the expert's process or techniques are based on the methods and procedures of science rather than on subjective belief or unsupported speculation.

The courts have articulated many criteria by which qualification of the expert and reliability of the opinion may be judged. Although expressed in different ways, similar rules are applied in the federal state courts.

Usually the first comprehensive exposure a lawyer or a judge will have to an expert's opinion is through his or her report. It is at this point that Greenfield and Gottschalk address the role of the forensic psychiatrist, advising how to prepare an effective psychiatric report. The authors assume that the preparers of these reports are qualified as psychiatrists or other mental health experts, and they assume that the opinions are based on recognized principles of psychiatry. The purpose of the book is to suggest how to communicate these opinions and the reasons for them effectively.

The role that psychological/psychiatric factors play in resolving a wide range of legal problems can hardly be overemphasized. This book is a guide to the preparation of reports that may shape the lives and fortunes of individuals and upon which the safety of the community will often depend. During approximately 26 years in private practice and 28 years as a federal trial judge, I have relied (or not relied) on many hundreds of such reports. One example illustrates the three time frames that Greenfield and Gottschalk address.

A young man entered Fort Dix and with a knife eviscerated his mother, an army sergeant. Successive psychiatric reports addressed (1) the past: What brought this now defendant to this point in his life, and was he not guilty by reason of insanity? (government and defense psychiatrists found he was not guilty by reason of insanity); (2) the present: Should this person be civilly committed? (not surprisingly, government and defense psychiatrists recommended civil commitment); (3) the future: Has this person's psychiatric treatment rendered him safe to be released to a halfway house or the community? (Psychiatric reports differed from time to time in their recommendation.)

As the authors explain, "[T]he term 'forensic' was meant to include information that assisted the courts of justice, or the 'forum' of justice." The book provides many examples of criminal and civil issues in which forensic psychiatry is of indispensable assistance to the courts, but a principal contribution is its guidance in the manner in which a civil and criminal forensic psychiatric report should be prepared for clarity and ease of communication. By way of example, numerous criminal and civil reports are included. Were these formats to be followed generally, the tasks of lawyers and judges would be greatly facilitated and the judge's gatekeeping function would be eased.

Most intriguing are the summaries and opinions of a number of criminal and civil psychiatric reports that are included in this volume. They are enlightening because they illustrate the wide range of subjects that forensic psychiatry must address. In the criminal field this includes the insanity defense, competency to stand trial, the risk of repeat sex offense, and intoxication. In the civil field, forensic psychiatry extends to questions of ability to return to work, depression, posttraumatic stress disorder, posing danger in the workplace, appropriate treatment of psychiatric disorder, foreseeability of repeat sexual offenses, mental competency to manage affairs, mental competency to execute a will, competency to carry on a profession, and contract duress.

These summaries are informative not only because they suggest the range of subjects that forensic psychiatrists must address; they are intriguing because they provoke the reader to decide if he or she would reach the same opinion that is arrived at in the example. Each example summarizes very briefly the problem presented and then sets forth the opinion of the psychiatrist. Of course, the summaries provide only the barest information, and the opinions were hardly based solely on such a limited foundation. But in a number of instances the reader can enjoy second-guessing the opinion.

Although forensic psychiatrists and other mental health professionals will be the primary beneficiaries of this book, lawyers and judges will also benefit from it.

Dickinson R. Debevoise, Senior USDJ
Newark, New Jersey
June 2008

Preface

In Chapter 1 ("Modelling English") of his wonderful and arcane *The Cambridge Encyclopedia of the English Language* (1995), the author, Professor David Crystal, gives the following six answers to the question, "Why study the English language?": "Because it's fascinating . . . important . . . fun . . . beautiful . . . useful . . . there" (Crystal, 1995, p. 3).

We contend that all of these reasons apply to this volume—to writing effective forensic mental health expert reports—and for the following reasons:

- "Because it's important." As the Honorable Dickinson R. Debevoise, Senior USDJ, points out in his foreword to this volume, "Usually the first comprehensive exposure a lawyer or a judge will have to an expert's opinion is through his or her report." Given that fact, given that first impressions are lasting ones, and given the potential usefulness of forensic reports in negotiating and arriving at resolutions of cases, these reports are *important* and should be well structured, well reasoned, and well presented.

- "Because it's fascinating." Both authors of this volume have commented to friends and colleagues innumerable times over the years that we "don't make these stories up. We couldn't. They're too weird . . . Truth is stranger than fiction." Many of the stories—the history underlying the cases presented in this volume—make for *fascinating* reading, and have the additional benefit of being true.

- "Because it's fun." This goes along with "Because it's fascinating." For the forensic mental health expert (whether psychiatrist, psychologist, or any other stripe) who likes to write, recording in written form the fascinating tales that the expert learns in consulting a particular case is not only important and required for the consultations, but it's *fun* and *useful,* as described next.

- "Because it's useful." As lawyers so often say, "If it isn't in writing, it didn't happen," and as prehistorians and historians point out, the written record has enabled humanity to proceed from generation to generation without having to reinvent the wheel every 30 years or so (Feder, 2004). In forensic mental health experts' roles in legal cases, the act of organizing information and thoughts and presenting them persuasively not only provides a potentially *useful* negotiating tool, but is also *useful* in helping counsel and the expert prepare for testimony (at trial, deposition, or hearing) in cases that go that far.

"Because it's beautiful." While it may be a stretch to say that any given forensic report ranks with Shakespeare or Hemingway as a literary work of art, a well-written report should certainly tell a good story, and may well be the basis for a *beautiful* work of literary art later on. Indeed, in the case of this volume, the authors hope that its readers find these stories interesting and compelling, if not beautiful.

■ "Because it's there." Finally, as a practical matter, many jurisdictions and venues require a written record—a report—of the forensic experts' findings, impressions, and opinions as part of the litigation process. The expert may not want to have to write such reports, and may prefer other aspects of the litigation process, such as testifying. But often, if a written report for the litigation record is not produced, the expert may not be part of the game. Forensic reports are *there*, as an integral part of the litigation process.

We have written this volume as a handbook, with multiple examples of reports and parts of reports, to assist the neophyte, novice, apprentice (trainee), reasonably experienced, and very experienced forensic mental health practitioner with forensic expert report writing.

In the first chapter of this book ("The Importance of Forensic Reports"), we present a rationale and proposed structure and format for clear, detailed, and persuasive report writing, recognizing that such reports are and should be clinically based. We also present a taxonomy of criminal and civil types of cases in which forensic mental health experts may be called to consult. We assert that the usefulness of persuasive forensic expert reports may occur from the very beginning of the expert's consultation (negotiation between counsel in the pre-indictment phase in criminal matters and in the pretrial phase in both criminal and civil matters) to the end of that consultation (testimony at hearing or trial), or anywhere in between (at deposition testimony, for example). We draw an analogy between the expert's written report and trial counsel's *trial notebook* (a collection of records, materials, and documents, with commentary, for use at trial, in guiding counsel through the various phases of a trial). The expert's written report is an effective way of helping the testifying expert organize anticipated testimony and keep track of records, materials, and other such documents to which referral may be needed during testimony.

Chapter 2 ("Forensic Reports and the Law") presents a brief overview of the history, goals, and (most important) evidentiary aspects of English and American common law relevant to the forensic mental health expert. This chapter is not intended as an "Introduction to Western Law," or "A Summary of Everything You've Learned in Three Years of Law School in the United States," or the like, but rather as a brief discussion of the rationale and scope of the use of forensic psychiatric/psychological information, input, and opinions—offered through mental health professionals qualified as experts—in the legal process. The reader should consult with counsel (which is *always* strongly advised) on any given case, and/or with any of a number of legal and forensic treatises, tests, journals, and so forth (as listed, for example, in Appendices B1, B2, and B3 of this book) to expand their database of the basic legal concepts presented in this chapter.

Using the format suggested in Chapter 1, numerous full criminal reports of actual cases, fictionalized and redacted for privacy and confidentiality purposes, illustrative of the points raised and discussed in Chapter 1, are provided. We walk the reader through the several steps and parts of these reports with discussion of each part in the context of the full report. We conclude with the "Summary and Opinions" of the forensic mental health expert's evaluation in each case. By following the chronological format and flow of such a report, both the forensic expert, and counsel or court, can comprehend the expert's findings, impressions, and opinions effectively and concisely at all phases of the expert's involvement in the case, pretrial, and at trial (if the case goes that far). We begin each full case with a case overview to familiarize the reader with the salient features of the case, and we conclude each full case with a commentary to review the important points made in the report from the forensic mental health perspective.

Following from Chapter 3 ("Full Criminal Reports"), Chapter 4 ("Criminal Summaries") gives a series of redacted and fictionalized "Summary and Opinions" sections of forensic psychiatric/psychological reports dealing with such topics in criminal law as reduced criminal responsibility (legal insanity, diminished capacity, intoxication), competency to stand trial, and others. These discussions are keyed to the types of criminal law psychiatric evaluations presented in Table 1.2 ("Criminal Issues as the Subject of Forensic Mental Health Evaluations and Reports").

Next, in Chapter 5 ("Full Civil Reports") we present numerous complete civil reports of actual cases also fictionalized and redacted, and also illustrative of the points raised and discussed in Chapter 1. As with Chapter 3, we provide a case overview for each full report; walk the reader through the several steps and parts of the report with discussion of these steps and parts; conclude the report itself with the "Summary and Opinions" section of the forensic psychiatrist's evaluation in the case; and give a commentary of the salient points and opinions of the forensic mental health expert. As with the criminal reports in Chapter 3, by following the chronological format and flow of this report, the forensic expert, counsel, and the court can comprehend the expert's findings, impressions, and opinions effectively and concisely at all phases of the expert's involvement in the case, pretrial, and at trial (again, if the case proceeds that far).

Like Chapter 4 for criminal matters, Chapter 6 ("Civil Summaries") presents a series of redacted and fictionalized summaries and opinions on forensic mental health expert reports. These reports deal with such topics in civil law as professional liability (medical malpractice), psychiatric effects in personal injury and workplace sexual harassment materials, civil competency to handle one's affairs, and other civil topics that forensic mental health experts are often asked to evaluate. As in Chapter 4, these discussions are keyed to the types of civil law psychiatric evaluations given in Table 1.3 ("Civil Issues as the Subject of Forensic Mental Health Evaluations and Reports") of Chapter 1.

Finally, Chapter 7 is the epilogue for this book. In it, we reiterate the rationale and salient areas addressed in this volume, emphasizing the importance of the written report in many aspects of a forensic mental health practice and in the related forensic mental health activities of forensic mental health experts.

The several appendices of this book consist of (a) a glossary of acronyms used in forensic mental health practice that are used in this book (Appendix A); (b) lists of four sets of references and suggestions for further reading in forensic mental health areas, presented in four appendices (B1, B2, B3, and B4): (i) books and monographs in forensic mental health, (ii) selected periodicals in this field, (iii) useful Web sites in this field, and (iv) selected professional literature references concerning report-writing in forensic mental health practice; and (c) Appendix C, entitled "Adjunctive Use of Tests, Inventories, Surveys, and Other Instruments and Assessment Tools in Forensic Mental Health Evaluations," discussing the instruments and assessment tools used in many of the cases and reports in this book.

Daniel P. Greenfield, MD, MPH, MS
Jack A. Gottschalk, JD, MA, MSM
Millburn, New Jersey
June 2008

References

Crystal, D. (1995). *The Cambridge encyclopedia of the English language.* Cambridge: Cambridge University Press.

Feder, K. L. (2004). *The past in perspective: An introduction to human prehistory* (3rd ed.). New York: McGraw-Hill.

Acknowledgments

Both authors acknowledge the help and encouragement of friends and colleagues over the years too numerous to list. Dr. Greenfield particularly thanks his students, professional colleagues and friends, attorneys, judges, and administrators who have referred cases and advised and consulted with him over the years, and the many individuals whom he has evaluated and sometimes treated over the years, who have made up what might be termed his experiential database for this book.

We both also thank Judge Debevoise for his insightful foreword to our book; the Springer Publishing Company (especially Sheri Sussman, senior vice president, editorial, who has been an exacting but realistic and delightful taskmistress in the publishing process, and her assistant, Deborah Gissinger) for taking on this project and moving it from an idea to a book; and to Tara LeGates, Dr. Greenfield's principal manuscript typist, who put the book's words into print.

Introduction

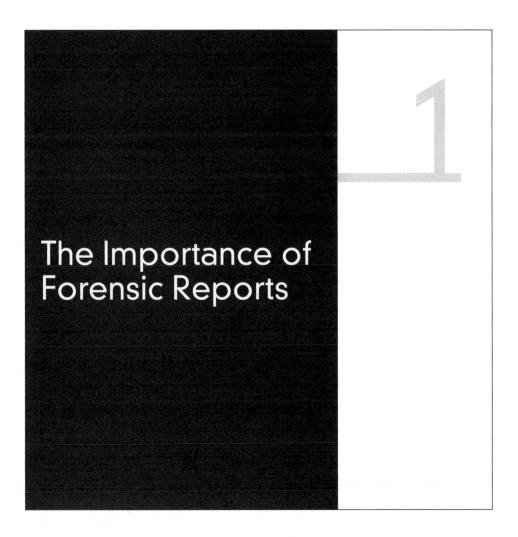

The Importance of Forensic Reports

Why read (or write) a book specifically about writing forensic reports?

In forensic (unlike clinical) mental health practice, one of the two main products created is the report containing the evaluation of the individual or topic on whom or on which the legal case is based. The other product—not nearly as common as the written report—is live or videotaped testimony at trial, hearing, or deposition. Each of these will be further discussed.

Returning, however, to the written report, the evaluating (forensic) mental health professional (typically a psychiatrist, psychologist, or social worker) must generally prepare a written opinion report about the forensic psychiatric/neuropsychiatric/addiction medicine/other issues involved in the case evaluation. That report is a critical and primary element in terms of the forensic practitioner's participation in the case. By contrast, for the clinical surgeon, for example, the operative report and hospital discharge summary are secondary to the surgical procedure and treatment themselves. These reports are necessary for documentation, statistical, and medicolegal purposes, and (in our experience) are often considered a necessary evil by most surgeons who must prepare them.

For the mental health professional, reports are also vital because of the wide range of cases with which they must deal in terms of forensic consultation. These cases are clearly far greater in terms of number and variety than is true in other medical specialties, and involve such diverse subjects as mental state, motivation, emotional condition, and other psychological/psychiatric factors.

In criminal law, for example, the forensic mental health clinician is generally asked to address issues that go to the heart of the alleged offender—the *mens rea* (evil intent)—in terms of mental state and psychiatric/neuropsychiatric/ addiction medicine condition during one (or more) of three time frames: the past, the present, and the future. These time frames will be discussed now.

- *The past:* This time frame is explored with regard to which of the criminal responsibility-reducing defenses (as of the time of the offense) may potentially be available to the defendant: legal insanity, diminished capacity, intoxication, or variants of these. Additionally, the question may be raised in criminal forensic mental health evaluations of whether the alleged offender, when first interrogated by law enforcement authorities, was competent to waive or surrender constitutionally guaranteed rights against self-incrimination (*Miranda* rights) as provided under the Fifth Amendment.
- *The present:* This time frame is concerned with the individual's involvement with the legal process, that is, when pretrial motions, trial, plea negotiations, and related matters are under way. Here such issues as competency to stand trial or to proceed to trial, or a determination of potential dangerousness, are the major considerations.
- *The future:* Once a criminal case has been resolved, such issues as "future dangerousness" of the adjudicated offender often arise, for example, after a finding of not guilty by reason of insanity. At that point, the placement of the individual must be addressed. Depending on the underlying criminal offense, this can mean placement in a highly restrictive and secure setting, such as a high-security psychiatric hospital. In the case of individuals who (after completion of their custodial sentences for sex offense convictions) are civilly committed as sexually violent predators (SVPs), or sexually dangerous persons (SDPs), their "likely" or "highly likely" potential to reoffend sexually is an example of the future dangerousness question that forensic mental health professionals are often asked to address. Addressing it, of course, requires a civil commitment to a high-security setting for treatment and concurrent isolation from society.

Table 1.1 presents these time frames and associated forensic psychiatric/ neuropsychiatric/addiction medicine evaluations in criminal law, in a graphic format.

Turning to civil law, forensic mental health evaluations, in our experience, generally address two areas in which inferences about evaluated individuals' underlying mental state and psychiatric/neuropsychiatric/addiction medicine conditions are relevant to the case at hand. These correspond largely to the *past* and *present* time frames in criminal law, and include the following

1.1	Time Frames for Criminal Forensic Psychiatric Evaluations	

Past	Present	Future[a]
At time of investigation	Competency to stand trial/ proceed to trial	Competency to stand trial/ proceed to trial Dangerousness
▓ Legal insanity	Civil commitment (present dangerousness)	▓ Civil commitment (involuntary psychiatric hospitalization)
▓ Diminished capacity	▓ Sex offenders	▓ Sexual civil commitment (sexually violent predator [SVP]/sexually dangerous person [SDP])
▓ Intoxication	▓ Civil commitment (involuntary hospitalization)	▓ Outpatient registration of sex offenders ("Megan's Law")
▓ Other committees		▓ Outpatient civil commitment ("Kendra's Law" in New York)
At time of offense		
▓ *Miranda* rights waiver		

[a]For the "reasonably foreseeable future." An unpublished consensus among about 35 superior court judges in New Jersey, from an informal poll conducted on November 21, 2006, agreed with a time frame of weeks-to-months—in contrast to other time frames such as days-to-weeks, or months-to-years—for this standard of "reasonably foreseeable future." Otherwise, the authors of this book, the 35 polled superior court judges, and numerous other researched sources do not define a more specific time frame for this standard.

applications: (a) the *past:* as of the time an individual entered into a contract, consented to an invasive medical procedure, made a will, or otherwise engaged in activities requiring the cognitive ability to have done so in an informed and knowing way; and (b) the *present* and *future:* as of the time of an individual's mental health evaluation, in terms of that individual's response to a physical or psychological injury (such as from an automobile or slip-and-fall accident; from alleged sexual harassment or wrongful discharge from a job; and from alleged toxic workplace exposures, to name only a few examples).

In some instances, both criminal and civil aspects of the same case may be issues in different matters pertaining to the same facts and circumstances. In the famous case, for example, of *California v. O. J. Simpson,* Simpson was found not guilty of criminal charges using the applicable criminal standard "beyond a reasonable doubt" likened to 95%, the burden of which to prove is borne by the state. However, based on the same facts in a later civil case, Simpson was found liable for civil charges by a jury, using the lower "preponderance of the evidence" standard likened to 51%—a civil standard of proof, the burden also to be borne by the plaintiff.

Once the forensic mental health professional's report is done, it may be used by counsel or the court in negotiating, as a basis for different types of motions, or as bases for the professional's testimony at a deposition, hearing, or trial, if testimony occurs in the case. In the first two contexts, a well-reasoned and persuasively written report can be extremely useful in the negotiating and motion practice process. In the last context, the professional's report can be useful in testimony, as a guide to testimony, and for reference to records reviewed. The structure of forensic reports, as well as these elements in reports, will be discussed at length later in this chapter.

The Subject Matter

Pulling together the points about the nature and types of forensic issues that can be the subject of forensic mental health evaluations and reports, Table 1.2 and Table 1.3 list examples of these issues in criminal and civil law, respectively, presented by the subject matter of the legal issues involved.

1.2 Criminal Issues as the Subject of Forensic Mental Health Evaluations and Reports

Traditional Criminal Responsibility-Reducing Psychiatric Defenses:
- Legal insanity
- Diminished capacity
- Intoxication
- Irresistible impulse

Sex Offenses
- Sex offenses
- Sexually violent predators (SVPs)/Sexually dangerous persons (SDPs)
- Community notification (Megan's Law registrants)

Domestic Violence
Malingering
Arson
Competency to Stand (Proceed to) Trial
Mitigation issues (death penalty)
Embezzlement
Battered Woman (spouse) Syndrome (syndrome evidence cases)
Blackouts
Elder Abuse

Future Dangerousness
- *Miranda* (constitutional rights) waiver
- Mitigation of penalty (federal sentencing guidelines)
- Suicide
- Transfer (waiver; referral issues for juveniles)

1.3 Civil Issues as the Subject of Forensic Mental Health Evaluations and Reports

- Employment law (sexual harassment; discrimination; others)
- Personal injury (including sexual abuse)
- Professional liability (malpractice)
- Mental health law (civil commitment, including SVPs/SDPs)
- Toxic exposure
- Professional regulation
- Will contests
- Dram-shop liability
- Competency (civil)
- Divorce
- Custody and visitation

The common thread of all of these types of evaluations pertains to the assessment of psychiatric and psychological aspects of individuals who have committed (or who may commit) offenses, or have been involved in traumatic situations, whether civil, criminal, or familial. These aspects, may, in turn, pertain to the individual's mental state (cognitive capacity, emotional state, motivation, or other such psychiatric/psychological factors) at the three different periods of time presented in Table 1.1 for criminal matters, for civil matters, and for matters including overlap between the two.

The Structure of This Book

In the course of 20-plus years of psychiatric practice, the first author of this volume (Dr. Greenfield) has been called on to evaluate hundreds of individuals in forensic contexts, has examined almost all of them, has prepared detailed reports on almost all of those actually seen, and has testified (at trial, hearing, or deposition) in many of those cases. Whether or not those cases were resolved or settled before the evaluating mental health professional's testimony was taken, the importance of the forensic report in these cases cannot be underestimated.

In our experience, notwithstanding the extensive technical literature in forensic mental health, practical materials specifically concerning writing clear and persuasive forensic mental health reports are lacking. To address this dearth of material in this important aspect of forensic mental health practice, we offer this text as a practical handbook for approaching and writing clear, useful, and persuasive forensic mental health reports.

We have divided this book into four major sections:

1. In the first section we present basic information about both the nature and scope of mental health evaluation reports, and the law. We specifically intend

to give an overview of the principles and practice of forensic mental health issues and of the law for the readers of this book who are mental health professionals at all levels of training and experience.

2. In the second section of this book, beginning with Chapter 3, we present numerous full-length criminal reports that illustrate several types of criminal matters in which forensic mental health evaluations may be done. Each of these reports is preceded by a brief case overview summarizing the case and describing its salient features. We then guide the reader on a step-by-step basis through the report parts, showing how each section of the report is constructed, and how the professional opinion of the evaluator is presented in the report (Chapter 3). We conclude each report with a case analysis and outcome and a discussion of forensic aspects of the cases. This analysis is intended to convey to the reader how the report served in helping to resolve its case.

    In Chapter 4, we then present examples of reports summarized from the summary and opinions (Table 1.4) sections of the actual reports, corresponding to the types of cases listed in Table 1.2.

    Following the criminal case summaries, we continue the format of the second section of the book, by presenting several full-length civil reports, showing on a step-by-step basis how the report is done (Chapter 5). As with the criminal chapter (Chapter 3), each case is preceded by a case overview and followed by a case analysis and outcome.

    In Chapter 6, we present a number of sample reports, summarized from the "Summary and Opinions" (Table 1.4) sections of the actual reports, corresponding to the types of cases listed in Table 1.3.

3. In the third section, the epilogue, we reiterate a number of salient points previously raised in the text that bear repetition and reinforcement. These include such practical points as explicitly articulating and listing, or describing, the forensic mental health issues to be addressed in the evaluation and report; writing the report in a clear, direct, and succinct way; using jargon-free language and avoiding psychobabble; and other such take-home practical points.

4. Finally, in the last section of the book, we present three appendices that supplement materials in the body of the book. These appendices are:
    A: Glossary
    B: References
        1: Books and monographs
        2: Journals and periodicals
        3: Internet resources
        4: Supplemental materials concerning the nature, scope, purpose, and writing of forensic reports.
    C: Assessment Tools Discussions of frequently used psychological, chemical dependency, and related tests, inventories, surveys, and other such instruments used in forensic mental health practice.

We recognize how bewildering the vocabulary and acronyms used by mental health professionals can be, especially to those not accustomed to their use. To assist the reader in that area, the glossary (Appendix A) defines acronyms commonly used.

The Reports

Next, a few words on the format of the reports presented in this book are in order.

The format for most of the reports in this book is derived from clinical report formats, such as hospital discharge summaries, in which the individual evaluated is presented as a clinical case starting with the identifying information (including forensic issues to be addressed), then proceeding through the clinical history, to the mental status/psychiatric examination (including testing), to diagnostic considerations, and finally to a discussion of the forensic mental health opinion(s) of the evaluator in response to the forensic issues presented early on in the report. Table 1.4 summarizes this format. (We are referring here to those reports involving clinical evaluations of living persons, but obviously not involving will contest evaluations or other *caveat* proceedings, and not necessarily involving dram-shop cases.) Appendix B4 presents references and articles specifically about forensic report writing.

Throughout the book, we use the same format for each of the eight full reports. That format involves (a) a brief introduction to the report through a capsule summary (case overview) of the case and of the forensic mental health issues addressed in the report; (b) the full report itself, following the full or modified clinically based format described in Table 1.4; and (c) a commentary following each full report, reviewing and highlighting the forensic mental issues raised and addressed in the report.

Essential Communication Skills With Counsel

At this early point, we list a series of practical pointers that have evolved during the authors' practices and collaboration on this book. We will make periodic references to these pointers throughout the book, and will recapitulate them at the end of the book, in the epilogue.

The importance of these pointers, we believe, is that if they are carefully and consistently followed by forensic mental health practitioners, counsel, and the courts who retain these practitioners, the interaction, communication, and

---

1.4 Format of Forensic Reports

I. Introduction (evaluation questions; records reviewed)
II. History (past history; history of the forensic incident and its aftermath; family history)
III. Mental Status/Psychiatric Examination (including psychological/chemical dependency testing)
IV. Clinical Diagnostic Impressions (in *Diagnostic and Statistical Manual of Mental Disorders, Fourth Edition, Text Revision,* or *DSM-IV-TR* format)
V. Summary and Opinions (responses to evaluation questions; psychiatric/psychological/neuropsychiatric/addiction medicine opinions)

cooperation among all of these professionals will be easy, productive, efficient, and harmonious. These pointers are:

- Maintain contact with other professionals involved in the case. In our experience, it is rarely true that too many cooks spoil the broth. Ongoing professional cooperation and communication are always a plus.
- Always be ready to listen to other views. Nobody has a monopoly on knowledge. The acquisition of knowledge and new and different perspectives, and the vetting of new ideas, are all activities encouraged among experts, retaining counsel, and the courts.
- Be attentive. Focus on the subject at hand. Despite the modern interest in multitasking, its value is not always practical or professional. For the forensic mental health practitioner, there must be only one point of focus, which must be the individual(s) being evaluated, and the forensic mental health issues raised in that evaluation.
- Avoid unnecessary delays and take responsibility for them if they occur. Appointments must be kept on time, reports provided with care and diligence, and all other responsibilities fulfilled. But, bad things do happen. When they do, admit to them, and learn from them.
- Communicate clearly. Avoid clouding of communication with needless professional jargon. Think about how your communication will be received and perceived by the intended audience, even if that audience is only one person. Make messages simple with as little room as possible for misunderstanding and obfuscation.
- Return telephone calls and related communications promptly. You must assume that when someone calls you, e-mails you, or otherwise communicates with you, that person believes it was important and necessary to do so. Within reason, close the communications gap and return the call as soon as possible. If a particular mode of communication is not to your liking (such as e-mail), make your communication preference clear to others at the beginning of your professional relationship, and try to accommodate your communicator's preference as well.
- Time is precious. Don't waste it. Time management is a skill that comes more easily to some than to others. Wasting time costs resources, both your own and those of others in the professional community. Spend some time learning to manage it.

In Conclusion

We conclude this introductory chapter with two caveats.

First, this volume is intended to be a practical, hands-on book about writing clear and persuasive forensic mental health reports. It is not written as a scholarly or technical treatise on the subject. To address the needs of readers for more theoretical and technical information about forensic mental health issues, Appendices B1–B4 list selected articles, books, and Internet sites that the authors have found useful and informative over the years. The reader is referred to these works for further information and for questions raised by the cases presented in this volume. Beyond that, we do not cite specific references, cases, or other such documentation referable to specific cases and issues presented.

Second, we acknowledge that forensic mental health reports can be written effectively and usefully in many different ways. Here we present one approach to forensic mental health report writing by reviewing sets of examples that have been useful for one particular practitioner of forensic psychiatry. We do not intend to suggest that these samples are the *only* way to structure and write forensic mental health reports. Rather, we do suggest that these sample reports reflect an effective, useful, and tried-and-true approach to that essential aspect of forensic mental health practice, the writing of clear, persuasive, and compelling reports. Appendix B4 lists a number of articles and references that discuss the writing of forensic mental health reports.

Conveying to the reader the importance of the written mental health expert report in the forensic arena, and helping that reader to write clear, persuasive, and compelling reports are the two major goals of our book.

Forensic Reports and the Law

Forensic psychiatric reports serve the essential and primary purpose of providing assistance in the resolution of both criminal and civil cases. This chapter explores and reviews some elements of the law that these reports are designed to serve. Clearly, this information is not intended to be a replacement for a course in law any more than reading about medicine would lead to actual medical practice. However, this chapter will provide a valuable package of information to social workers, mental health professionals, and others who will need to understand the law and its relationship to their activities.

We start by exploring the definition of *forensic,* an exploration that is easier to attempt than to complete with specific accuracy. In a broad and historic sense, the term *forensic* was meant to designate information that assisted the courts of justice, or the *forum* of justice. While that is still true, that word now applies to specific disciplines, including forensic accounting, forensic medicine, forensic anthropology, and almost any other imaginable kind of specialized undertaking applicable to legal concerns. Forensic psychiatry, as a branch of forensic medicine, is our target here.

Medicine, of course, often plays a major role in the courts, with probably the most recognized action (in the eyes of the public) being that of the medical examiner who determines the cause of death of a victim in a homicide case.

By contrast, the forensic mental health practitioner is asked to do clinically based evaluations, to prepare reports, and (often) to offer expert professional testimony concerning the mental state of a defendant in a criminal case. In civil matters, the forensic psychiatrist is tasked with the responsibility, perhaps less dramatic (depending on the case) but equally critical, of evaluating for competency, and the characterizing psychological result (that is, damages) of crimes, workplace incidents, personal injuries, and so forth. The professional training and expertise of the forensic mental health practitioner may be needed by prosecutors and defense lawyers in criminal cases, by plaintiffs and defendants in civil matters, and by the court as an aid in the resolution of any case. Mental health practitioners may be retained to do evaluations by any of these three "players" in the criminal and civil legal systems.

Having set out the need for mental health evaluations and reports in the wide range of legal issues, it is now necessary to examine those two main systems, criminal and civil, which together constitute the law as we know it.

The Criminal Law

The criminal law encompasses not only the wide range of acts that are defined as crimes under federal and state law, it also encompasses pretrial detention, trial, sentencing, probation, and supervised release. Forensic psychiatry may have a role not only in determining whether a crime has been committed, but also at each of these other stages of criminal proceedings.

It was recognized early in the development of modern civilization (which, for our purposes, we shall consider as that of England) that some acts were of such a heinous character (*malum in se,* or "bad in themselves") that there was no need even to codify them. The common law thus recognized seven acts (burglary, arson, rape, robbery, mayhem, murder, and sodomy) that were classified as felonies (high crimes) and thus punishable by forfeiture of lands and property, or by death.

While we neither intend nor desire in this chapter to create a treatise on law and society, these felonies were, in some cases, particularly relevant both to those times and to the present. Arson, for example, was greatly feared because of the close-knit living of the populace and fire-prone construction of virtually every structure save, of course, for stone castles. Mayhem, defined generally as the malicious cutting off of a limb, was of significant importance in an age in which self-defense and hunting were activities that required functioning limbs.

Written laws at that time, as might be expected, grew to be far more in number. The acts that these laws addressed were described as being *malum prohibitum,* translated to mean "wrong because prohibited." These offenses, while also felonies, often called for less severe penalties, even as is true today. They included (to name only a very few) larceny, embezzlement, criminal assault, daytime burglary, and literally hundreds of other acts. A less serious grouping of crimes were classified as misdemeanors. These crimes generated less severe penalties upon conviction. They are also with us today.

In modern times, the use of other terms to describe felonies and misdemeanors has, in some jurisdictions, been adopted for reasons that are, at best, obscure, and at worst, confusing. In New Jersey, for example, until that state adopted a criminal code in 1979, felonies were known as high misdemeanors, and misdemeanors as misdemeanors. The state now punishes offenders under a criminal code that contains first-, second-, third-, and fourth-degree crimes.

By whatever name, crimes in general must involve intent on the part of the offender, that is, a *mens rea* or guilty mind. The question of whether and when such intent existed in the past, exists at present, or will exist in the future (see Table 1.1 in Chapter 1) is one in which the practice of forensic psychiatry with the attendant reports is of high importance. Within this context, the forensic psychiatrist aids the criminal justice system in helping to determine whether or not a defendant, based on past, present, or future conditions, can interpose a defense based on legal insanity, diminished capacity, involuntary intoxication, passion provocation, or irresistible impulse, depending on the law in a particular jurisdiction.

The Civil Law

Unlike the criminal law that seeks to punish offenders for wrongs that are deemed to have been committed against society (i.e., the state), the civil (sometimes called private) law seeks to regulate and resolve legal issues that arise from contracts, torts (civil wrongs), family domestic relations, wills, and other noncriminal matters. The end result of such disputes is money damages or, in some cases, injunctive relief in which a party is compelled to do something or not to do something.

In addition to the differences between the basic goals of the criminal and civil law, there are also significant procedural differences that can vary from jurisdiction to jurisdiction. These include (depending on the jurisdiction) smaller jury sizes in civil (as opposed to criminal) cases; the need for a unanimous jury vote in a criminal case compared to a majority vote in civil matters; and the standard of proof needed for resolutions "beyond a reasonable doubt," in a criminal case, and only by "preponderance of the evidence" in many civil cases and "clear and convincing evidence" in certain other civil cases, such as civil commitment of mentally ill and dangerous individuals.

Despite these procedural and substantive differences between criminal and civil cases, the role of the forensic psychiatrist can be just as important in a civil case as in a criminal one. Determination of a person's competence or of psychological injury, the causation of a psychiatric impairment, and whether a person acted intentionally all can have critical consequences in the outcome of a civil case.

Again, while the role of the forensic psychiatrist in a civil matter is often less dramatic than in a criminal one, the importance of that role is in no way less critical. The types of civil cases in which forensic psychiatry is often consulted by lawyers and sometimes by the court are many (see Table 1.3 in Chapter 1).

Standards for Expert Testimony

The need for expert testimony in helping to resolve both civil and criminal cases is wide-ranging, reaching into virtually every area where specialized knowledge is needed to assist a jury or, in a bench trial, a case heard by a judge alone. It is generally believed that the use of expert testimony first occurred in 1782. As society and the issues that went before the courts became more complex, the need for expert testimony grew ever more important.

In the United States, the standards for the acceptance of expert testimony varied somewhat among the state jurisdictions until 1923 when the federal case of *Frye v. U.S.* was decided by the U.S. Court of Appeals for the District of Columbia. In shorthand terms, the *Frye* decision established the standard that expert scientific testimony was admissible as evidence if it was generally accepted within the scientific community. The standard was thus established in the federal system and the state courts.

The *Frye* standard, however, was radically changed by the United States Supreme Court in *Daubert v. Merrill Dow,* in 1993. In that case it was held that the hearsay safeguard under Federal Rules of Evidence made such a strict approach to admissibility unnecessary and that a more flexible standard was needed that would put the trial courts in a position to determine, on a case-by-case basis, if the expert testimony is scientifically reliable and helpful to the fact-finding process. The result of these decisions is that *Daubert* became the standard in all federal courts. At the state level, some states have adopted *Daubert* and others have retained *Frye.*

The Ultimate Goal

Whether the forensic psychiatrist is called upon to use professional training and experience to help resolve either a criminal or civil case, whether called upon to do so by counsel or by the court itself, the ultimate goal is the same. The principal, persistent, and underlying consideration is the requirement to assist the legal system in its attempts to achieve a fair and just resolution to the case.

The Reports

3

Full Criminal Reports

In this chapter, we present a series of four full-length forensic criminal psychiatric reports, modified and redacted to protect privacy, following the format described in Chapter 1. These reports constitute a representative sample of the types of criminal cases a forensic mental health expert would be likely to encounter in consulting to attorneys (prosecution or defense) or to the courts. They include:

- Intoxication (Voluntary)
- Competency to Stand Trial
- Malingering
- Child (Sexual) Abuse

After guiding the reader through the deconstructed reports with boldface commentary and discussion, we reproduce one of the four civil reports *(State v. Edward Taylor Hard)* in full to give the reader a full picture of the final report.

State v. Edward Taylor Hard

Case Overview: Intoxication (Voluntary)

The following full case report is based on an incident that took place in a bar where a voluntarily intoxicated individual, and the defendant, Edward Taylor Hard, shot and killed another individual with whom the defendant had a prior negative relationship. Counsel for the defendant, Priscilla Proctor, Esquire, retained a psychiatrist, Abel D. Fence, MD, MPH, because of his combined background, training, and credentials in psychiatry, neuropsychiatry, pharmacology, and medicine, to evaluate the defendant.

In presenting the report, we will deconstruct and discuss each part of it, and walk the reader through the report, section by section. This format of the report follows that described in Chapter 1, Table 1.4. Dr. Fence's report follows.

The Report

In the first section of the report, the writer lays out the nature and scope of the report, and the issues to be discussed in it. This introduction is brief and concise. It makes reference to specific questions asked and issues raised by retaining defense counsel, even to the point of quoting excerpts of defense counsel's initial letter of engagement (which presents the issues to be addressed and terms and parameters of the consultation, including financial; in that sense, that initial letter may be considered a contract, of sorts, between counsel and the forensic expert).

Following up on our telephone discussions and correspondence about the above-captioned matter, and based upon the sources of information listed below, I am writing you this report. This report is provided at your request to address my medical/pharmacologic/toxicologic/neuropsychiatric opinion—held with a degree of reasonable medical probability—about Mr. Edward Taylor Hard's state of mind and state of intoxication, if applicable, during the period of time in question when he shot Mr. Bruno Summers in what appears to have been a bar brawl during the evening (approximately 10:00 P.M.) on September 3, XXXX, with his own pistol.

In the interest of saving time, and since the records, materials, and other sources of information in connection with this matter are extensive and detailed with regard to the actual events of the slaying, subsequent law enforcement investigations, autopsy findings of Mr. Summers, and toxicologic data (about both Mr. Hard and Mr. Summers), I will not reiterate those details.

Rather, after briefly reviewing Mr. Hard's history leading up to the incident in question, especially with regard to his history of alcoholism and substance abuse, I will focus on Mr. Hard's state of intoxication and state of mind during the evening in question, as indicated above, and will also focus on my clinical neuropsychiatric/toxicologic findings, impressions, and opinions that bear most closely on the reasons for which this evaluation was requested.

Again, as expressed in your letter of transmittal of January 21, XXXX, those reasons pertain to "your analysis of my client's state of intoxication and state of mind during the time of the shooting incident at the Unicorn Tavern in which Mr. Bruno Summers was killed. I am particularly interested in your professional opinions about the applicability of an intoxication, insanity, diminished capacity, or 'irresistible impulse' legal test in this matter, and I am taking the liberty of forwarding to you under separate cover statutory, case, and other such materials concerning those defenses" (excerpted, in part, from your letter of transmittal of January 21, XXXX).

In the next section of the report—still the introduction—the writer presents and discusses the sources of information on which the report is based. As described in Chapter 1, these sources generally boil down to written records and materials (often including DVDs and videos); the clinically based interview/examination of the subject; adjunctive testing (Appendix C); collateral interviews of significant others (such as parents, friends, witnesses, etc.); and the forensic expert's own collection of data and areas of expertise specific to the case at hand, if applicable.

With the above background and introduction, the sources of information upon which this neuropsychiatric/toxicologic evaluation and report are based are as follows:

1. My review of the packet of discovery materials provided to you by the Office of the Prosecuting Attorney in this matter (subsequently forwarded to me by your office), as well as police investigation reports, witness statements, photographs and drawings of the crime scene, toxicologic studies of Mr. Summers and Mr. Hard, documentation concerning Mr. Hard's ownership of the murder weapon, medical records about Mr. Summers from Mercy Hospital, Dr. Dorian Flannery's [Medical Examiner] autopsy report of Mr. Summers, newspaper articles concerning the shooting incident, and other such records and materials.

2. My neuropsychiatric/toxicologic interview/examination of Mr. Edward Taylor Hard at Jamner County Correctional Center on January 31, XXXX, in an interview room, which interview/examination included the administration and subsequent scoring of a series of standardized and unstandardized psychological, chemical dependency, and related tests and inventories, as described below.

3. As part of my neuropsychiatric/toxicologic evaluation of Mr. Hard, the administration and subsequent scoring of a series of standardized and unstandardized psychological and chemical dependency tests and inventories, as follows:

   a. The Minnesota Multiphasic Personality Inventory, 2nd edition, or MMPI-2;
   b. The Millon Clinical Multiaxial Inventory, 3rd edition, or MCMI-III;
   c. The Beck Depression Inventory, 2nd edition, or BDI-II;
   d. The Michigan Alcohol Screening Test, or MAST;

e.   The Drug Abuse Screening Test, or DAST;
f.   The Alcohol Use Disorders Identification Test, or AUDIT;
g.   The Addiction Assessment survey instrument (unstandardized);
h.   The Past Medical History (unstandardized) survey form;
i.   The Cognitive Capacity Screening Examination, or CCSE; and
j.   The Mini-Mental State Examination, or MMSE.

4.   My telephone discussions/interviews with Ms. Debra Summers (Mr. Bruno Summers's widow); Mr. James Goodhart (Mr. Hard's drug and alcohol counselor from several of his inpatient and outpatient alcohol detoxification and rehabilitation treatment programs); Reginald B. Wonder, DO (Mr. Hard's family physician for about the past 25 years); Ms. Jane Whitehair (Mr. Hard's retired sixth grade teacher at the Everett Elementary School in New, Major); Mr. Eustace ("Easy") Hard (Mr. Hard's father); Ms. Neva ("Never") Hard (Mr. Hard's mother); and Ms. Sophie ("Softie") Hard Grobanofski (Mr. Hard's oldest sister).

5.   My knowledge, background, training, and experience in medicine, pharmacology and toxicology, psychiatry, and neuropsychiatry.

The next major section of the report—like that of a clinical consultation report—presents and discusses the history of the events that led to the forensic mental health issue in the case, beginning with the earliest background and history ("Personal History," "Past History," "Family History," etc.). As in clinical consultation reports, this pre-incident background gives the reader an understanding of what in the evaluee's life led to the incident at issue, and when applicable, how and why in a psychological or psychodynamic formulation the offense took place.

History

Mr. Edward Taylor Hard is a 28-year-old single (never married) childless white male, originally from a rural area (Neva, Major), more recently from Ruston, and currently incarcerated in the Jamner County Correctional Center in connection with charges of murder in the first degree arising from his having shot Mr. Bruno Summers in the chest at point-blank range during what appears to have been a bar brawl at the Unicorn Tavern (in Ruston) at about 10:00 P.M. on September 3, XXXX. Mr. Hard is a self-employed painter (which he describes having been the case for about two years prior to the shooting incident). He also describes a long-standing history of alcoholism (primarily) and drug abuse (secondarily) since he was about 11 years of age. He was raised in what he described as a dysfunctional and alcoholic family situation and background for all of his life.

With regard to Mr. Hard's *past history* and *past psychiatric history*, as just described, he presents a history in a general sense of a difficult, alcoholic, and dysfunctional family situation. He is the third-youngest in a sibship of 11, with his next-older brother, Kevin (approximately 14 months older than Mr. Hard himself) having died of an overdose of alcohol and Placidyl at the age of 14 (when Mr. Hard himself was in the sixth grade).

Mr. Hard attended local schools in Neva, Major, for most of his years of formal education (he dropped out of high school at age 16, in the 10th grade, after staying back for two years), having been sent to a local military academy (the Fortress, in Marine Corps, Major). He had to leave that school during the seventh grade because of financial problems in meeting tuition payments. Mr. Hard described himself as an "average student," but one who "got into trouble a lot" (his words) for various disciplinary reasons, including those related to his criminal history (described below and elsewhere in available records and materials).

Mr. Hard's parents, Eustace and Neva Hard, were a hardware store clerk and a housewife and homemaker, respectively, both of whom had serious drinking problems; seriously dysfunctional and conflictual family situation, and histories of having physically and sexually abused all of their children "at one time or another" (Mrs. Hard's words). This abuse occurred especially while their children were young (both Mr. and Mrs. Hard deny any legal repercussions of this abusive and incestuous activity). Mr. Edward Hard himself, by his description, resorted to alcohol and drug abuse at an early age "to escape from my family" (his words), and, as a result, described in only vague terms incidents and episodes in his childhood, his schooling, and so forth. He engaged in sexual activities at an early age, both heterosexual and homosexual, describing a period of uncertainty about his sexual preference when he was in his late teens and early 20s. He finally "settled for a woman" (his words) when he was about 22 years of age. He dated a succession of women, and among others, lived for a relatively long period of time (about 6 to 8 months, by his recollection) with Ms. Debra Flathead Summers (Mr. Bruno Summers's widow), which period of cohabitation ended approximately two years prior to the shooting incident. In this regard, it is significant in my opinion that Ms. Summers had two pregnancies, reportedly, by Mr. Hard, and that she independently and without his knowledge or agreement terminated both pregnancies.

Up to this point, Mr. Hard's dysfunctional and difficult childhood and adolescence have been emphasized, foreshadowing his ongoing and more serious later problems. This exemplifies the clinically informed nature of the report, and enables the writer to develop the theme of psychopathology from a wide variety of sources, leading to the offense in question.

Following his leaving high school at age 16, Mr. Hard held a succession of jobs of a manual nature, including working as a gas station attendant, a landscaper, an auto mechanic assistant, and other such positions. He made efforts to pass his General Educational Development (GED) test over about a four-year period, concluding at about age 22, but without passing his GED, explaining (to me, during my interview/examination of him) that "I got fed up . . . I found I didn't need it."

Again, without reviewing details, the above summarized Mr. Hard's dysfunctional, alcoholic, and marginal life and existence for virtually his entire life, and presents a backdrop to the shooting that occurred in the evening of September 3, XXXX; that incident will be described below.

> At this point in this particular case, events specifically related to the incident in question are discussed. These events involved the same type of incident as the offense at issue in this case, and are an important additional piece of information to the evaluation and report.

With regard to the shooting incident of September 3, XXXX, the events associated with that incident are as follows. In late August, XXXX, shortly before Bruno and Debra Summers were married, Mr. Hard and Mr. Summers met and had an altercation at the Unicorn Tavern (please see above records for details). A long-standing animosity had existed between the two individuals for a number of years, partly due to Mr. Hard's previous relationship with Mrs. Summers and partly due to his repugnance at Mr. Summer's activities and role as a leader of a local survivalist neo-Nazi organization.

As a result of this altercation, Mr. Hard sustained injuries to his teeth and lip (after Mr. Summers punched him), and commented at the time in a threatening way toward Mr. Summers. Mr. Hard denied any other contact with Mr. Summers from that time to the time of the shooting incident, so that the next contact the two men had was on the evening of that shooting.

> By this point in the "History" section of the report, the stage has been set to present and discuss the incident in question. That follows next.

During the evening of September 3, XXXX, Mr. Edward Hard was a patron at the Unicorn Tavern, a bar that he had frequented often for many years. Mr. and Mrs. Bruno Summers (who had been married for about two [2] weeks at that point) came to the tavern after dinner (according to Mrs. Summers's account). Mr. Summers took exception to Mr. Hard's perceived advances toward his wife, and confronted Mr. Hard in what was described as an aggressive manner. Mr. Hard, remembering his previous encounter with Mr. Summers (from August, XXXX), became frightened, vaguely perceived a threat to himself, pulled his gun, and shot it, intending to shoot the wall and not Mr. Summers. However, the bullet did strike Mr. Summers in the left chest, knocking him over. Chaos ensued in the tavern, and medical assistance was obtained for Mr. Summers. He was transported to Mercy Hospital, where emergency room triage and subsequent treatment, and later treatment in the intensive care unit (according to the medical examiner's report and Mercy Hospital records) of pneumonia induced by the gunshot wound (GSW) to his chest, were administered. Mr. Summers's condition worsened, and he succumbed to that pneumonia after four days of hospitalization.

> At this point in the report, the shooting incident took place, and is described through the eyes of the shooter. The next part of the report provides some commentary about Mr. Hard's perceptions and anticipates Dr. Fence's forensic psychiatric/neuropsychiatric/addiction medicine opinions, as presented and discussed in the "Summary and Opinions" section of the report.

What specifically happened after the shooting incident at the tavern was not clear from available records and reports. However, subsequent police investigation led to Mr. Hard's home, where he initially denied having been at the Unicorn Tavern at the time of the shooting (he indicated that he had been drinking beer and watching TV at home). However, Mr. Hard subsequently acknowledged that he had been, in fact, present at the tavern at the time, and that he was the individual who had shot Mr. Summers. He cooperated with police officers in their investigation (e.g., by showing them the murder weapon in his apartment). Mr. Hard was arrested for the death of Mr. Summers, and his subsequent criminal processing included breathalyzer testing of Mr. Hard's blood alcohol concentration (BAC) performed at 005 hours (12:05 A.M.), approximately three (3) hours after the actual shooting (according to the Jamner Police Department Alcohol Influence Report). At that testing, Mr. Hard's BAC was 0.16% where 0.10% is the legal threshold for driving while intoxicated (or DWI) in the State of Major. Implications of these findings will be discussed below.

Following that processing, Mr. Hard was transferred to the Jamner County Correctional Center (JCCC), where he remains incarcerated at the present time, pending the outcome and disposition of his case.

> Also in keeping with the clinically based format described in Chapter 1, the next section of the report presents observations and findings from the psychiatric/neuropsychiatric/addiction medicine perspective, relevant to the evaluation.

Mental Status (Psychiatric) Examination

Mr. Edward Taylor Hard, as described above, was seen in an interview room at the JCCC. I introduced myself to him, ascertained his understanding of the purpose and scope of the interview/examination, and advised him of the likelihood nonconfidential nature of the evaluation. He told me this was acceptable to him. We then proceeded with the interview/examination.

Mr. Hard presented as a slight, sallow, thin, well-developed white male whose eye contact was limited and whose overall demeanor appeared depressed and lackluster. He was casually groomed and dressed in JCCC attire, and wore jogging shoes. He had a heart-shaped tattoo on the lateral surface of his left biceps with the words "Ed and Deb" (referring to Mrs. Debra Summers) positioned underneath the heart. His speech was unremarkable with regard to language, flow, and rhythm, although he appeared to show a great deal of remorse and regret about the incident. On several occasions, he expressed a strong psychological attachment and even a preoccupation with Mrs. Summers (his former girlfriend, as noted above, and the woman who had been pregnant by him twice).

> Since forensic mental health evaluation may not be confidential or privileged between the evaluator and the evaluee, it is important to point that out to evaluees at the beginning of the interview/examination, and to obtain their permission and consent to proceed. Some mental health professionals (like this writer) obtain such written consent with a formal instrument, analogous to obtaining informed consent to medical or surgical procedures; others do not. In criminal defense cases, it is ultimately defense counsel who decides whether the defense expert's opinion and report will be used, as an extension of a defendant's "right to remain silent." In prosecution-retained and court-appointed forensic mental health evaluations, in contrast, the defendant, in effect, has waived his or her privilege in previously offering a psychiatric defense, which may be explored by a prosecution and/or court-appointed expert. Therefore, no privilege or confidentiality applies to the evaluation and report, which are then made available to the defense, the prosecution, and the court.

With the exception of the depressed and fatigued overall demeanor, there was no indication during this interview/examination of severe affective disorder (such as depression, mania, or suicidality), or of thought disorder/psychotic processes (such as hallucinations, delusions, loosening of associations, and so forth). Cognitively, Mr. Hard was alert and oriented in all parameters (time, person, place, and circumstances of and reasons for this interview/examination). His responses on the two above-noted cognitive screening tests (i.e., the Mini-Mental State Examination, or MMSE, and the Cognitive Capacity Screening Examination, or CCSE) did not indicate any organicity or cognitive impairment, and his overall presentation was consistent with his level of education and life experience, in my opinion.

Mr. Hard's responses to the above-noted psychological and chemical dependency tests and inventories indicated a considerable degree of psychopathology

> The point to be emphasized here is that as of the time of Dr. Fence's interview/examination, there were no mental status (psychiatric) examination findings indicative of clinically significant mental abnormalities. Although this observation would not have had any direct bearing on inferences about Mr. Hard's underlying mental state and psychiatric/neuropsychiatric/addiction medicine condition in terms of his criminal responsibility for the shooting, it is important with regard to Mr. Hard's psychiatric condition at the time of the interview/examination by Dr. Fence, and in that way, in terms of his "competency to stand trial" status at that time, and for the reasonably foreseeable future after that.

and psychiatric disturbance, and also confirmed his history of long-standing and serious chemical dependency problems (especially alcoholism), as also indicated above. For further details of these findings, and of this information, please refer to the above-listed psychological, medical, and chemical dependency tests, inventories, and surveys.

Leading up to the "Summary and Opinions" section of the report, this next section summarizes the evaluator's diagnostic impressions of the person evaluated, again from a clinical perspective. These impressions are presented in *DSM-IV-TR* terminology and format. As a practical matter, the *DSM-IV-TR* is so widely used and acknowledged as an authority in the mental health professions (including the forensic mental health professions) that the mental health professional is well advised to use that schema, and not others, for forensic reports.

Clinical Diagnostic Impressions

In keeping with the current diagnostic nomenclature and format of the *Diagnostic and Statistical Manual of Mental Disorders, Fourth Edition, Text Revision* (2000), of the American Psychiatric Association, clinical diagnostic impressions for Mr. Hard can be presented as follows:

Axis I (Clinical Disorders):

1. Polysubstance dependence, in institutional remission.
2. Dysthymia.

Axis II (Personality Disorders):

Dependent personality disorder.

Axis III (General Medical Conditions):

Mr. Hard appears to be in generally good health, without indications of active, acute, chronic, or ongoing medical problems or conditions requiring medical attention or treatment, notwithstanding his long history of polysubstance dependence.

Axis IV (Psychosocial and Environmental Problems):

Mr. Hard's main present "Psychosocial and Environmental Problem," in my view, pertains to his "Problems related to the legal system/crime," in connection with his present charges, and prospects for further punishment. In addition, "Occupational problems" (limited experience and training), "Economic problems" (resulting from his occupational problems), and "Problems related to primary support group" (limited support and prospects) in an individual with chronic drug and alcohol abuse problems and chronic depression, in my opinion, apply here.

Axis V (Global Assessment of Functioning [GAF]):

A GAF Scale score of 60–70 signifying mild-to-moderate impairment and symptomatology, in my opinion, applies here.

The last section of the report—"Summary and Opinions"—is the most important part of the report, practically speaking, because it pulls together the preceding information and data in a concise and coherent way, presents the evaluator's "bottom line" forensic expert opinion about the central forensic issue(s) in the case, and in our experience is generally the first (and sometimes only) part of a report read by the retaining attorney or court. As such, this section needs to be a brief, pithy condensation of all of the preceding sections, and a persuasive statement of the forensic mental health expert's opinion in the case.

Summary and Opinions

Mr. Edward Taylor Hard is a 28-year-old single (never married) white male, unemployed (formerly a self-employed painter), who is currently incarcerated at the Jamner County Correctional Center (JCCC) pending the outcome and disposition of his current criminal case. Mr. Hard has a long-standing history of psychiatric disturbance and alcoholism, and was involved in an incident during the evening of September 3, XXXX, during which he shot Mr. Bruno Summers in what appears to have been a barroom brawl. In that vein, with that history, and in view of Mr. Hard's blood alcohol concentration (BAC) (0.16%) approximately three hours after the actual shooting, your office contacted me to do this neuro-psychiatric/toxicologic evaluation of Mr. Hard with respect to issues pertaining to possible legal defenses (including legal insanity) potentially available to him; specifics of your request are described above. The sources of information upon which this evaluation is based, as well as the findings and clinical impressions, are presented above and will not be repeated here.

At this point in this section, the author begins a discussion of the analysis of the several clinical-scientific areas on which the author's forensic expert opinions are based. For presentation purposes, each area is discussed in a separate paragraph, starting with (a) toxicologic issues, followed by (b) cognitive and addictive issues, and concluding with (c) personal background and family issues. Expert opinions are given in each of these paragraphs for each of the issues raised in the paragraphs.

From the toxicologic perspective, a consideration in this context assumes accepted principles of toxicology. These principles include a peak in Mr. Hard's alcohol absorption curve approximately one hour after the ingestion of his last drink; a burn-off rate and an accumulation postabsorption curve for Mr. Hard of 0.015%–0.020% per hour; and no additional alcohol intake by Mr. Hard after the actual time of the shooting. With the assumptions, Mr. Hard's extrapolated blood alcohol concentration (BAC) as of the time of the shooting would have been approximately 0.190% to 0.200%.

Then, taking into account Mr. Hard's dysfunctional and alcoholic family history; his prior history of an intimate relationship with Mrs. Debra Summers; his prior history of animosity with Bruno Summers; and his BAC at the time of the actual incident itself (0.190% to 0.200%), it is my neuropsychiatric/toxicologic opinion that Mr. Edward Taylor Hard's mental state would have been extremely confused and chaotic. This confusion and chaotic state was so severe that he was not able to think rationally, clearly, with intent, knowingly, purposefully, or in a goal-directed way at the time of the shooting of Mr. Bruno Summers.

In addition, considering Mr. Hard's prior dependent relationship upon Mrs. Summers and his animosity toward Mr. Summers, it is my opinion that at the time he saw the two of them together in the bar, he was unable to resist the impulse to engage in a confrontation with Mr. Summers to "rescue Debbie from that Nazi" (as he described his thinking during that period of time, in discussion with me during my interview/examination). When that confrontation "turned ugly" (his words again), whether that was actually the case or not, Mr. Hard reacted in a self-protective and self-defensive way, given the perceived threat and given his confused and intoxicated mental state at the time, so that he was simply unable to resist those impulses to protect and defend both Mrs. Summers and himself.

> Next, the author draws a connection between clinical findings and impressions and criminal/legal concerns pertaining to the defendant's criminal responsibility in this matter, as well as to potentially available psychiatric and related criminal responsibility-reducing defenses for the defendant. This connection, or link, between clinical and legal issues is the crux of the forensic consultation, and needs to be clearly, concisely, and persuasively written. The paragraph follows.

Finally, with regard to the legal questions of legal insanity and diminished capacity, as I understand those concepts, while Mr. Hard's state of intoxication and confused and addled thinking at the time of the incident were not so extreme, in my opinion, as to put him in the position of simply not knowing the nature and quality of the act in which he was engaged at the time, it is my opinion that his state of intoxication and confusion did negate an element of the offense, namely his ability to have acted knowingly and purposely in the shooting of Mr. Bruno Summers. Put more simply, in my professional opinion, held with a degree of reasonable medical probability, Mr. Edward Hard's intoxicated mental state during the period of time in question (of his shooting of Mr. Bruno Summers) would support a legal determination and defense of irresistible impulse, intoxication, and diminished capacity. It would not, in my opinion, support a legal determination of legal insanity.

> Last, Dr. Fence writes the customary disclaimers, distinguishing his forensic report from a purely clinical one.

The referenced individual was examined with reference to specific circumstances emanating from the incident in question, in accordance with the restrictive rules concerning an independent medical examination. It is, therefore, understood that no treatment was given or suggested, and that no doctor/patient relationship exists.

I aver that the information contained in this document was prepared by the undersigned and is the work of the undersigned. It is true to the best of my knowledge and information, and has not been modified by anyone other than the undersigned.

Please advise me if you have questions about this evaluation and report, or if you anticipate requiring additional services from me in connection with this matter.

Thank you very much.

Abel D. Fence, MD, MPH

Case Analysis and Outcome

Referring to Table 1.1, this evaluation focuses on Dr. Fence's inferences about the alleged perpetrator's underlying mental state and psychiatric/neuropsychiatric/ addiction medicine condition during a discrete period of time in the *past,* specifically at the time he allegedly shot the victim in this matter. Dr. Fence ultimately offered the expert opinions supporting criminal responsibility-reducing psychiatric defenses for the slaying, that is, irresistible impulse (not an accepted defense in all jurisdictions), intoxication (voluntary, in this case), and diminished capacity (a widely accepted defense). He also specifically offered an opinion that did not support one potentially available psychiatric defense, that is, legal insanity.

Dr. Fence was not asked to provide—and did not offer—an opinion about another potential forensic mental issue in the past, that is, the defendant's mental competency to have "knowingly, voluntarily, and intelligently" waived his Constitutional *(Miranda)* rights not to give a statement, or confession during the early stage of police investigation of the slaying. Dr. Fence also did not offer (and was not asked) expert opinions about "Present" (Table 1.1, specifically "Competency to Stand Trial") or "Future" (Table 1.1, specifically "Competency to Stand Trial") or "Future" (Table 1.1, specifically future dangerousness)—forensic mental health time frame issues. In so doing, Dr. Fence focused his evaluation and report on specific forensic mental health issues requested by retaining defense counsel.

Periodically, the ethical issue for a forensic mental practitioner arises in which retaining counsel either does not raise forensic consultation issues that the consulted expert believes should be raised, or in which defense counsel specifically requests that such issues not be raised by the consulted expert. In both situations—which must, in our view, be assessed on a case-by-case basis—the differing advocacy positions of counsel (for the client) and the expert (for the opinions about the client) are underscored.

Dr. Fence prepared his report as a way chronologically to catalogue and review material and testify, if necessary, similar to the manner in which litigating attorneys prepare what may be termed a trial notebook.

This particular case was resolved through plea negotiations (defense counsel and prosecuting counsel, later approved by the court) without the necessity for trial or expert testimony by Dr. Fence. However, retaining defense counsel advised Dr. Fence prior to sentencing that his evaluation and report were instrumental in counsel's pressing the "diminished capacity" and "intoxication" defenses, and in negotiating a shorter custodial sentence for his client.

What follows is the full forensic expert's report, to give the reader an accurate picture of the final report, as submitted to retaining counsel or to the court.

Full Report

Cecil Davidson, Esquire
Davidson & McElroy
123 Main Street
Anytown, ST 12345
RE: State v Edward Taylor Hard
Indictment No.: 05-I-12386
Dear Mr. Davidson:

Following up on our telephone discussions and correspondence about the above-captioned matter, and based upon the sources of information listed below, I am writing you this report. This report is provided at your request to address my medical/pharmacologic/toxicologic/neuropsychiatric opinion—held with a degree of reasonable medical probability—about Mr. Edward Taylor Hard's state of mind and state of intoxication, if applicable, during the period of time in question when he shot Mr. Bruno Summers in what appears to have been a bar "brawl" during the evening (approximately 10:00 p.m.) on September 3, XXXX, with his own pistol.

In the interest of saving time, and since the records, materials, and other sources of information in connection with this matter are extensive and detailed with regard to the actual events of the slaying, subsequent law enforcement investigations, autopsy findings of Mr. Summers, and toxicologic data (about both Mr. Hard and Mr. Summers), I will not reiterate those details.

Rather, after briefly reviewing Mr. Hard's history leading up to the incident in question, especially with regard to his history of alcoholism and substance abuse, I will focus on Mr. Hard's state of intoxication and state of mind during the evening in question, as indicated above, and will also focus on my clinical neuropsychiatric/toxicologic findings, impressions, and opinions that bear most closely on the reasons for which this evaluation was requested.

Again, as expressed in your letter of transmittal of January 21, XXXX, those reasons pertain to "your analysis of my client's state of intoxication and state of mind during the time of the shooting incident at the Unicorn Tavern in which Mr. Bruno Summers was killed. I am particularly interested in your professional opinions about the applicability of an intoxication, insanity, diminished capacity, or 'irresistible impulse' legal test in this matter, and I am taking the liberty of forwarding to you under separate cover statutory, case, and other such materials concerning those defenses" (excerpted, in part, from your letter of transmittal of January 21, XXXX).

With the above background and introduction, the sources of information upon which this neuropsychiatric/toxicologic evaluation and report are based are as follows:

1. My review of the packet of discovery materials provided to you by the Office of the Prosecuting Attorney in this matter (subsequently forwarded to me by your office), as well as police investigation reports, witness statements, photographs and drawings of the crime scene, toxicologic studies of Mr. Summers and Mr. Hard, documentation concerning Mr. Hard's ownership of the murder weapon, medical records about Mr. Summers from Mercy Hospital, Dr. Dorian Flannery's [Medical Examiner] autopsy report of Mr. Summers, newspaper articles concerning the shooting incident and other such records and materials);

2. My neuropsychiatric/toxicologic interview/examination of Mr. Edward Taylor Hard at Jamner County Correctional Center on January 31, XXXX, in an interview room, which interview/examination included the administration and subsequent scoring of a series of standardized and unstandardized psychological, chemical dependency, and related tests and inventories, as described below;

3. As part of my neuropsychiatric/toxicologic evaluation of Mr. Hard, the administration and subsequent scoring of a series of standardized and unstandardized psychological and chemical dependency tests and inventories, as follows:

   a. The Minnesota Multiphasic Personality Inventory, 2nd edition, or MMPI-2;
   b. The Millon Clinical Multiaxial Inventory, 3rd Edition, or MCMI-III;
   c. The Beck Depression Inventory, 2nd Edition, or BDI-II;
   d. The Michigan Alcohol Screening Test, or MAST;
   e. The Drug Abuse Screening Test, or DAST;
   f. The Alcohol Use Disorders Identification Test, or AUDIT;
   g. The Addiction Assessment survey instrument (unstandardized);
   h. The Past Medical History (unstandardized) survey form;
   i. The Cognitive Capacity Screening Examination, or CCSE; and
   j. The Mini-Mental State Examination, or MMSE;

4. My telephone discussions/interviews with Ms. Debra Summers (Mr. Bruno Summers's widow); Mr. James Goodhart (Mr. Hard's drug and alcohol counselor from several of his inpatient and outpatient alcohol detoxification and rehabilitation treatment programs); Reginald B. Wonder, DO (Mr. Hard's family physician for about the past 25 years); Ms. Jane Whitehair (Mr. Hard's retired sixth grade teacher at the Everett Elementary School in New, Major);

Mr. Eustace ("Easy") Hard (Mr. Hard's father); Ms. Neva ("Never") Hard (Mr. Hard's mother); and Ms. Sophie ("Softie") Hard Grobanofski (Mr. Hard's oldest sister); and

5. My knowledge, background, training, and experience in medicine, pharmacology and toxicology, psychiatry, and neuropsychiatry.

History

Mr. Edward Taylor Hard is a 28-year-old single (never married) childless white male, originally from a rural area (Neva, Major), more recently from Ruston, and currently incarcerated in the Jamner County Correctional Center in connection with charges of "Murder in the First Degree" arising from his having shot Mr. Bruno Summers in the chest at point-blank range during what appears to have been a bar brawl at the Unicorn Tavern (in Ruston) at about 10:00 P.M. on September 3, XXXX. Mr. Hard is a self-employed painter (which he describes having been the case for about two years prior to the shooting incident). He also describes a long-standing history of alcoholism (primarily) and drug abuse (secondarily) since he was about 11 years of age. He was raised in what he described as a dysfunctional and alcoholic family situation and background for all of his life.

With regard to Mr. Hard's *past history* and *past psychiatric history*, as just described, he presents a history in a general sense of a difficult, alcoholic, and dysfunctional family situation. He is the third-youngest in a sibship of 11, with his next-older brother, Kevin (approximately 14 months older than Mr. Hard himself) having died of an overdose of alcohol and Placidyl at the age of 14 (when Mr. Hard himself was in the sixth grade).

Mr. Hard attended local schools in Neva, Major, for most of his years of formal education (he dropped out of high school at age 16, in the 10th grade, after staying back for two years), having been sent to a local military academy (the Fortress, in Marine Corps, Major). He had to leave that school during the 7th grade because of financial problems in meeting tuition payments. Mr. Hard described himself as an "average student," but one who "got into trouble a lot" (his words) for various disciplinary reasons, including those related to his criminal history (described below and elsewhere in available records and materials).

Mr. Hard's parents, Eustace and Neva Hard, were a hardware store clerk and a housewife and homemaker, respectively, both of whom had serious drinking problems; seriously dysfunctional and conflictual family situation, and histories of having physically and sexually abused all of their children "at one time or another" (Mrs. Hard's words). This abuse occurred especially while their children were young (both Mr. and Mrs. Hard deny any legal repercussions of this abusive and incestuous activity). Mr. Edward Hard himself, by his description, resorted to alcohol and drug abuse at an early age "to escape from my family" (his words), and, as a result, described in only vague terms incidents and episodes in his childhood, his schooling, and so forth. He engaged in sexual activities at an early age, both heterosexual and homosexual, describing a period of uncertainty about his sexual preference when he was in his late teens and early 20s. He finally "settled for a woman" (his words) when he was about 22 years of age. He dated a succession of women, and among others, lived for a relatively long period of time (about 6 to 8 months, by his recollection) with Ms. Debra Flathead Summers (Mr. Bruno Summers's widow), which period of cohabitation ended approximately two years prior to the shooting incident. In this regard, it is significant in my opinion that Ms. Summers had two pregnancies, reportedly, by Mr. Hard, and that she independently and without his knowledge or agreement, terminated both pregnancies.

Following his leaving high school at age 16, Mr. Hard held a succession of jobs of a manual nature, including working as a gas station attendant, a landscaper, an auto mechanic assistant, and other such positions. He made efforts to pass his General Educational Development (GED) test over about a four-year period, concluding at about age 22 without passing his GED, explaining (to me, during my interview/examination of him) that "I got fed up . . . I found I didn't need it."

Again, without reviewing details, the above summarized Mr. Hard's dysfunctional, alcoholic, and marginal life and existence for virtually his entire life, and presents a backdrop to the shooting that occurred in the evening of September 3, XXXX; that incident will be described below.

With regard to the shooting incident of September 3, XXXX, the events associated with that incident are as follows. In late August, XXXX, shortly before Bruno and Debra Summers were married, Mr. Hard and Mr. Summers met and had an altercation at the Unicorn Tavern (please see above records for details). A long-standing animosity had existed between the two individuals for a number of years, partly due to Mr. Hard's previous relationship with Mrs. Summers and partly due to his repugnance at Mr. Summers's activities and role as a leader of a local survivalist neo-Nazi organization.

As a result of this altercation, Mr. Hard sustained injuries to his teeth and lip (after Mr. Summers punched him), and commented at the time in a threatening way toward Mr. Summers. Mr. Hard denied any other contact with Mr. Summers from that time to the time of the shooting incident, so that the next contact the two men had was on the evening of that shooting.

During the evening of September 3, XXXX, Mr. Edward Hard was a patron at the Unicorn Tavern, a bar that he had frequented often for many years. Mr. and Mrs. Bruno Summers (who had been married for about two [2] weeks at that point) came to the tavern after dinner (according to Mrs. Summers's account). Mr. Summers took exception to Mr. Hard's perceived advances toward his wife, and confronted Mr. Hard in what was described as an aggressive manner. Mr. Hard, remembering his previous encounter with Mr. Summers (from August, XXXX), became frightened, vaguely perceived a threat to himself, pulled his gun, and shot it, intending to shoot the wall and not Mr. Summers. However, the bullet did strike Mr. Summers in the left chest, knocking him over. Chaos ensued in the tavern, and medical assistance was obtained for Mr. Summers. He was transported to Mercy Hospital, where emergency room triage and subsequent treatment, and later treatment in the intensive care unit (according to the medical examiner's report and Mercy Hospital records) of pneumonia induced by the gunshot wound (GSW) to his chest, were administered. Mr. Summers's condition worsened, and he succumbed to that pneumonia after four days of hospitalization.

What specifically happened after the shooting incident at the tavern was not clear from available records and reports. However, subsequent police investigation led to Mr. Hard's home, where he initially denied having been at the Unicorn Tavern at the time of the shooting (he indicated that he had been drinking beer and watching TV at home). However, Mr. Hard subsequently acknowledged that he had been, in fact, present at the tavern at the time, and that he was the individual who had shot Mr. Summers. He cooperated with police officers in their investigation (e.g., by showing them the murder weapon in his apartment). Mr. Hard was arrested for the death of Mr. Summers, and his subsequent criminal processing included breathalyzer testing of Mr. Hard's blood alcohol concentration (BAC) performed at 005 hours (12:05 A.M.), approximately three (3) hours after the actual shooting (according to the "Jamner Police Department Alcohol Influence Report"). At that testing, Mr. Hard's BAC was 0.16% where 0.10% is the legal threshold for driving while intoxicated (or DWI) in the State of Major. Implications of these findings will be discussed below.

Following that processing, Mr. Hard was transferred to the Jamner County Correctional Center (JCCC), where he remains incarcerated at the present time, pending the outcome and disposition of his case.

Mental Status (Psychiatric) Examination

Mr. Edward Taylor Hard, as described above, was seen in an interview room at the JCCC. I introduced myself to him, ascertained his understanding of the purpose and scope of the interview/examination, and advised him of the likelihood nonconfidential nature of the evaluation. He told me this was acceptable to him. We then proceeded with the interview/examination. Mr. Hard presented as a slight, sallow, thin, well-developed white male whose eye contact was limited and whose overall demeanor appeared depressed and lackluster. He was casually groomed and dressed in JCCC attire, and wore jogging shoes. He had a heart-shaped tattoo on the lateral surface of his left biceps with the words "Ed and Deb" (referring to Mrs. Debra Summers) positioned underneath the heart. His speech was unremarkable with regard to language, flow, and rhythm, although he appeared to show a great deal of remorse and regret about the incident. On several occasions, he expressed a strong psychological attachment and even a preoccupation with Mrs. Summers (his former girlfriend, as noted above, and the woman who had been pregnant by him twice).

With the exception of the depressed and fatigued overall demeanor, there was no indication during this interview/examination of severe affective disorder (such as depression, mania, or suicidality), or of thought disorder/psychotic processes (such as hallucinations, delusions, loosening of associations, and so forth). Cognitively, Mr. Hard was alert and oriented in all parameters (time, person, place, and circumstances of and reasons for this interview/examination). His responses on the two (2) above-noted cognitive screening tests (i.e., the Mini-Mental State Examination, or MMSE, and the Cognitive Capacity Screening Examination, or CCSE) did not indicate any organicity or cognitive impairment, and his overall presentation was consistent with his level of education and life experience, in my opinion.

Mr. Hard's responses to the above-noted psychological and chemical dependency tests and inventories indicated a considerable degree of psychopathology and psychiatric disturbance, and also confirmed his history of long-standing and serious chemical dependency problems (especially alcoholism), as also indicated above. For further details of these findings, and of this information, please refer to the above-listed psychological, medical, and chemical dependency tests, inventories, and surveys.

Clinical Diagnostic Impressions

In keeping with the current diagnostic nomenclature and format of the *Diagnostic and Statistical Manual of Mental Disorders, Fourth Edition, Text Revision* (2000), of the American Psychiatric Association, clinical diagnostic impressions for Mr. Hard can be presented as follows:

Axis I (Clinical Disorders):

1. Polysubstance dependence, in institutional remission.
2. Dysthymia.

Axis II (Personality Disorders):

Dependent personality disorder.

Axis III (General Medical Conditions):

Mr. Hard appears to be in generally good health, without indications of active, acute, chronic, or ongoing medical problems or conditions requiring medical attention or treatment, notwithstanding his long history of polysubstance dependence.

Axis IV (Psychosocial and Environmental Problems):

Mr. Hard's main present "Psychosocial and Environmental Problem," in my view, pertains to his "Problems related to the legal system/crime," in connection with his present charges, and prospects for further punishment. In addition, "Occupational problems" (limited experience and training), "Economic problems" (resulting from his occupational problems), and "Problems related to primary support group" (limited support and prospects) in an individual with chronic drug and alcohol abuse problems and chronic depression, in my opinion, apply here.

Axis V (Global Assessment of Functioning [GAF]):

A GAF Scale score of 60–70 signifying mild-to-moderate impairment and symptomatology, in my opinion, applies here.

Summary and Opinions

Mr. Edward Taylor Hard is a 28-year-old single (never married) white male, unemployed (formerly a self-employed painter), who is currently incarcerated at the Jamner County Correctional Center (JCCC) pending the outcome and disposition of his current criminal case. Mr. Hard has a long-standing history of psychiatric disturbance and alcoholism, and was involved in an incident during the evening of September 3, XXXX, during which he shot Mr. Bruno Summers in what appears to have been a barroom brawl. In that vein, with that history, and in view of Mr. Hard's blood alcohol concentration (BAC) (0.16%) approximately three hours after the actual shooting, your office contacted me to do this neuro-psychiatric/toxicologic evaluation of Mr. Hard with respect to issues pertaining to possible legal defenses (including legal insanity) potentially available to him; specifics of your request are described above. The sources of information upon which this evaluation is based, as well as the findings and clinical impressions, are presented above and will not be repeated here.

From the toxicologic perspective, a consideration in this context assumes accepted principles of toxicology. These principles include a peak in Mr. Hard's alcohol absorption curve approximately one hour after the ingestion of his last drink; a burn-off rate and an accumulation postabsorption curve for Mr. Hard of 0.015%–0.020% per hour; and no additional alcohol intake by Mr. Hard after the actual time of the shooting. With the assumptions, Mr. Hard's extrapolated blood alcohol concentration as of the time of the shooting would have been approximately 0.190% to 0.200%.

Then, taking into account Mr. Hard's dysfunctional and alcoholic family history; his prior history of an intimate relationship with Mrs. Debra Summers; his prior history of animosity with Bruno Summers; and his BAC at the time of the actual incident itself (0.190% to 0.20%), it is my neuropsychiatric/toxicologic opinion that Mr. Edward Taylor Hard's mental state would have been extremely confused and chaotic. This confusion and chaotic state was so severe that he was not able to think rationally, clearly, with intent, knowingly, purposefully, or in a goal-directed way at the time of the shooting of Mr. Bruno Summers.

In addition, considering Mr. Hard's prior dependent relationship upon Mrs. Summers and his animosity toward Mr. Summers, it is my opinion that at the time he saw the two of them together in the bar, he was unable to resist the impulse to engage in a confrontation with Mr. Summers to "rescue Debbie from that Nazi" (as he discussed his thinking during that period of time, with me during my interview/examination). When that confrontation "turned ugly" (his words again), whether that was actually the case or not, Mr. Hard reacted in a self-protective and self-defensive way, given the perceived threat and given his confused and intoxicated mental state at the time, so that he was simply unable to resist those impulses to protect and defend both Mrs. Summers and himself.

Finally, with regard to the legal questions of legal insanity and diminished capacity, as I understand those concepts, while Mr. Hard's state of intoxication and confused and addled thinking at the time of the incident were not so extreme, in my opinion, as to put him in the position of simply not knowing the nature and quality of the act in which he was engaged at the time, it is my opinion that his state of intoxication and confusion did negate an element of the offense, namely his ability to have acted knowingly and purposely in the shooting of Mr. Bruno Summers. Put more simply, in my professional opinion, held with a degree of reasonable medical probability, Mr. Edward Hard's intoxicated mental state during the period of time in question (of his shooting of Mr. Bruno Summers) would support a legal determination and defense of irresistible impulse, intoxication, and diminished capacity. It would not, in my opinion, support a legal determination of legal insanity.

The referenced individual was examined with reference to specific circumstances emanating from the incident in question, in accordance with the restrictive rules concerning an independent medical examination. It is therefore understood that no treatment was given or suggested, and that no doctor/patient relationship exists.

I aver that the information contained in this document was prepared by the undersigned and is the work of the undersigned. It is true to the best of my knowledge and information, and has not been modified by anyone other than the undersigned.

Please advise me if you have questions about this evaluation and report, or if you anticipate requiring additional services from me in connection with this matter.

Thank you very much.

Abel D. Fence, MD, MPH

State v. Theodore Princely

Case Overview: Competency to Stand Trial

This case involved an attempt to interview and evaluate a defendant, Theodore Princely, who was serving a life sentence for murder. While in prison, the defendant had escaped, had been recaptured, and had been returned to state prison. Defense counsel Malcolm Lambe, Esquire, sought a psychiatric evaluation to determine whether the defendant was competent to stand trial (CST) on the escape charge. Counsel retained Klaus Liebman, MD, MS, for that purpose. Dr. Liebman's report follows.

The Report

As in the *State v. Hard* report, in this one, the writer initially presents the nature, purpose, and scope of the report, and the issues to be discussed in it. However, in the interest of full communication with the retaining attorney (one of the pointers for an effective forensic practice, described in Chapter 1), recognizing that the actual interview/examination was curtailed, the writer discusses that issue at the very beginning of the report.

Following up on our telephone discussions and correspondence about the above-referenced matter, and based on the sources of information given below, I am writing you this report of my attempted psychiatric/neuropsychiatric/addiction medicine evaluation of Mr. Theodore Princely.

As you know, I use the word *attempted* because when I actually did make efforts to speak with Mr. Princely, he was located in his cell in the Administrative Segregation ("Ad Seg") Unit at Graito State Prison (GSP). He refused to speak with me, and at the very end of the brief attempt, he threw an odorless liquid at me through the crack in his cell door where the door meets the cell wall.

The Corrections Officer in charge (Captain Don Winslow) terminated the attempted interview after that. After completing a "Special Report" at the captain's request, I left GSP.

After describing the incomplete interview/examination, Dr. Liebman next discussed the inferences and conclusions that *could* be made on the basis of the terminated interview/examination.

What inferences about Mr. Princely's present (and anticipated future, as described below) mental state and psychiatric/neuropsychiatric condition that I can make based on that experience and on other sources of information in this matter (described below) will be the subject of this present report.

The writer then quoted extensively from retaining counsel's prior forensic communications to him, in order to focus on the specific forensic issues to be addressed in the evaluation and report.

By way of background and history of Mr. Princely in terms of this present evaluation, you requested in your transmittal letter (of criminal/discovery records and materials pertaining to this matter, discussed below) that I "evaluate Mr. Princely in order to determine whether he is competent to stand trial for the escape charge pending against him in the above entitled matter . . . I need to know whether you feel Mr. Princely is competent to proceed to trial and that he has the ability to participate in the presentation of his defense."

You also gave the following history of Mr. Princely's offenses, which led to this present evaluation:

Mr. Princely is serving a life sentence plus 10–12 years for a homicide. I believe he was a juvenile at the time and that the matter was waived up to adult court. I believe that he has been incarcerated for the past 27 years. Mr. Princely advises me that he was threatened by a man and told defendant he could "end up missing here and nobody would ever find you."

Mr. Princely took that as a death threat and one week later he left the prison. He was later arrested. In order to present a defense of duress or necessity he has to have tried to turn himself in to the authorities after he was safe from the threat that caused him to leave. Mr. Princely would not talk with me the last time I met and asked him to give me witnesses that could verify that he tried to turn himself in.

He rejected a four-year prison sentence to run concurrent with his present sentence, but would not tell why he was rejecting the offer despite the fact that he has no legal defense to the escape.

Prior to my last meeting with Mr. Princely, he has refused to talk with me via conference four times. He has acted out in court on a few occasions. The first time he suddenly went toward a sheriff's officer as if he were going to tackle him or go for his gun. On March 4, XXXX, Mr. Princely was shackled and surrounded by prison guards and without warning made a quick movement as if he were trying to get away. He was quickly taken to the ground.

I have been told by prison guards that the defendant is usually assaultive when he comes out of his cell and one guard thought he was on medication. Mr. Princely's acting out in court, his refusal to provide me with any defense witnesses, and his refusal to accept a good plea bargain where there appears to be no legal defense have caused me to question his fitness to proceed . . .

If, after your evaluation, you believe that Mr. Princely may have some type of psychiatric defense to the escape charge (i.e., suffering from some type of mental disease or defect), please advise me.

After giving the above introduction to the report, the writer next presents and discusses the sources of information on which the report is based. The records and materials are catalogued and summarized in such a way that the writer can use them in later testimony, if necessary, analogous to the attorney's use of a trial notebook (see Chapter 1) at trial.

With that background, the sources of information on which this present (limited) evaluation and report are based are as follows:

1. My review of copies of criminal/legal, medical, and other such records and materials provided to me by your office in connection with this matter, as follows:

   a. The statutory law on "Competency to Stand Trial" ("Mental Incompetent Excluding Fitness to Proceed . . . "), presenting and describing the elements and requirements for determination of an individual's CST status;

   b. The "Indictment" (No.: 96–01–00079-I/A; 01 Count, Third Degree, for Escape), stating that "THEODORE PRINCELY on or about the 8th day of July, XXXX, in the Township of Bonner, County of Wechsler . . . knowingly did without legal authority remove himself from official detention . . . "

   Supporting records and documentation gave details about Mr. Princely's escape, including a completed "Escape Notification/Identification Sheet" from the Riverbank State Prison (Farm) that "on July 1, XXXX at approximately 9:00 P.M. a formal count was taken at the Riverbank Farm and inmate Princely was unaccounted for. A recount confirmed that inmate Princely was missing and he was declared escaped at 9:45 P.M. . . . "

Other materials in this collection (specifically, a letter to you from Bruce Conway, Assistant Wechsler County Prosecutor, dated June 19, XXXX) indicated that Mr. Princely had been arrested in Los Angeles as an escapee, and "transferred back to and received at the State Prison at Bluntville on or about February 6, XXXX . . . "

In addition to these materials pertaining to Mr. Princely's escape, his "Criminal History Detailed Record" was included in this collection of records and materials; and

c. A collection of medical records and materials pertaining to Mr. Princely's evaluations and treatment in various correctional facilities (state prisons).

For present purposes, Mr. Princely's medical history is described in these records and materials as including asthma; a traumatic fracture (reportedly as the result of a fight) to his right hand in May of XXXX, with subsequent evaluations and treatment; and a closed head injury accident in April of XXXX (evaluated and treated at Briarcliff Medical Center in Bluntville, without consequences or sequelae, to my reading).

Medications prescribed over the years for Mr. Princely, as described in these records, have included Proventil inhaler (for his asthma), Motrin (a non-narcotic analgesic), and no psychotropic medications.

A psychological evaluation in August of XXXX (the month before Mr. Princely's escape) indicated that he had future plans, and hopes at that time to be together with his girlfriend and to get a job.

Those notes also reflect Mr. Princely's denial of any psychiatric history, including treatment, on his part.

Subsequent mental health notes (in XXXX, after Mr. Princely had been returned from his escape) described him as refusing to talk and as "hostile," with no mention made of any known (past or present) formal psychiatric diagnosis, history, treatment (including psychotropic medications), and so forth;

2. Our telephone discussion on July 5, XXXX, during which I elaborated on a previous voice-mail message I had left for you about my attempted interview/examination of Mr. Princely at the GSP, we discussed other aspects of this evaluation.

During that telephone discussion, to my direct question to you about whether or not in your opinion, Mr. Princely has the "ability to participate with [you] in an adequate presentation of his defense" (i.e., the last element of CST, according to the statute), you replied that he did not;

3. My attempt to do a psychiatric/neuropsychiatric interview/examination of Mr. Princely in his unit ("Ad Seg"; see above) at GSP, on June 5, XXXX. The course of that interview was described above. As a practical matter, because of Mr. Princely's refusal to speak with me, I did not obtain information about him from him, with the exception of my observing his withdrawn, angry, hostile, and uncooperative behaviors and demeanor (as described in further detail below); and

4. My knowledge, background, training, and experience in psychiatry and neuropsychiatry, addiction medicine, and forensic psychiatry.

Analogous to a clinical report (such as a "Discharge Summary"), the next section of the report ("History") gives a narrative account in chronological order of the background and history of the individual evaluated from the perspective of the issues to be addressed by the writer in this report. This approach also serves to orient both the writer and the readers (i.e., counsel, opposing counsel, and the court) to issues relevant to the writer's forensic evaluation.

History

Briefly, as I learned from records and materials, and from your initial transmittal letter of June 14, XXXX, Mr. Theodore Princely is a 38-year-old (DOB: April 5, XXXX), single, childless, African American male, originally from the Baltimore, Maryland, area, who was involved in an incident as a juvenile that resulted in his waiver to Superior Court on charges of homicide and armed robbery (details of the offenses in question are not available in the records provided to me for this evaluation).

Mr. Princely was convicted of those charges, sentenced to life imprisonment and 7 to 10 years. He is currently serving that sentence at GSP, as described above. For a period of about one and a half years, Mr. Princely was an escapee from incarceration, as also described above.

At this point, the writer shifts to a discussion of the events that led to this evaluation.

On July 1, XXXX, Mr. Princely escaped from the Riverbank State Prison (Farm), and remained away until he was arrested in Los Angeles (see above). He was then returned (on February 6, XXXX), where he has remained incarcerated in various State Department of Corrections (DOC) facilities.

As Mr. Princely's defense counsel for the charge relating to his escape from prison in XXXX, you arranged for this present (attempted) psychiatric/neuropsychiatric evaluation of Mr. Princely, to address issues about his CST status, specifically as described in your July 26, XXXX transmittal letter (see above).

In this context, I note Mr. Princely's lack of any formal history of psychiatric disorder or treatment (including psychotropic medications), as described in the medical records and materials from the DOC institutions (see above).

In addition to reviewing the criminal/legal and medical records and materials described above pertaining to Mr. Princely, this evaluation was to include a face-to-face interview/examination of Mr. Princely, including pencil-and-paper psychological, chemical dependency, and related testing [see Appendix C]. Arrangements were made for this interview/examination, including your arranging for an appropriate court order for my professional visit to the GSP.

> **Next, Dr. Liebman described the attempted interview/examination in step-by-step fashion.**

I went to the GSP for the interview/examination, where the staff was aware of the scheduled evaluation. I was taken by Captain Winslow to the Administrative Segregation Unit of GSP by the captain, and then taken to the area outside Mr. Princely's cell (Cell 283).

Captain Winslow did not want me to interview/examine Mr. Princely outside his cell, because as the captain told me, on recent previous occasions when Mr. Princely had been taken outside his cell, he refused to return, and acted out aggressively against the corrections officers who attempted to return him to his cell.

Initially, I sat in a chair that the Corrections staff brought to me outside Mr. Princely's cell, and observed him through the vertical slit window on the right side of his cell (Mr. Princely had this window taped over from the inside and from the bottom, for approximately three-quarters of the total length of the window. This left about 8–12 inches, by my estimate, for me to observe Mr. Princely).

I observed Mr. Princely, and noticed that he was a medium-height, medium-weight, well-developed African American male wearing the tan GSP outfit and a white towel on his head. Mr. Princely paced throughout his cell during my attempt to communicate with him, walking from his bed (on the far wall) to what appeared to be a sink (on the near wall, immediately adjacent to the door of his cell).

I spoke as loudly as I could to Mr. Princely, who mumbled words that I could not understand, and who gestured for me to move toward the other end of the door of his cell, the side of the door that opens to the outside when the cell is opened. I was aware of dull noises (which I thought were Mr. Princely speaking to me), and leaned over and bent down toward the side of the door in order to better hear Mr. Princely.

At that point, I was hit on the face, hair, and shoulders by a room-temperature odorless unknown liquid, which Mr. Princely had thrown at me through the crack in his cell door. Captain Winslow immediately terminated the interview, with my agreement, and I pulled away from the cell door. I went to the nursing station nearby, flushed out my face and my eyes with warm water, used soap on my face and eyes and hair and jacket, and then reflushed my face and my eyes.

The liquid stung briefly, but had no effects after I flushed and washed my face, hair, shoulders, and jacket.

After this incident, Captain Winslow and Sergeant Toune asked me to complete an incident report form ("Special Form"), which I did. You have a copy of that report from a previous communication, and another copy is attached.

As described above, this very limited interview/examination should not be considered complete. I would be willing to attempt to reinterview/examine Mr. Princely if you wish, although based on his behaviors and activities as reported

> At this point in the report, since this particular evaluation did not permit the writer to conduct a full "Mental Status/Psychiatric Examination," this particular report transitions into a combination of "Clinical Diagnostic Impressions" and "Summary and Opinions." The limitations of this report as well as reasonable inferences about Mr. Princely's competency to stand trial status are presented, with a straightforward opinion given about that issue. The question of malingering—almost always an issue in forensic practice—is addressed in a direct and straightforward way in this report, with the writer's noting that a psychiatric/neuropsychiatric opinion— held with a degree of reasonable medical probability—supports Mr. Princely's *not* being considered competent to stand trial, because of his lack of "Ability to participate with counsel in an adequate presentation of his defense."

to me by the corrections staff at GSP over at least the past several weeks to months, it is my professional opinion that it is extremely unlikely that such an attempt would be any more successful than this one.

> The next several paragraphs give the author's straightforward and direct forensic expert opinion about Mr. Princely's CST status, describing how observations and inferences of the incomplete interview/examination support the expert's opinion.

Taking into account all available sources of information, including my clinical observations and inferences about Mr. Princely's present underlying mental state and psychiatric/neuropsychiatric condition, as a practical clinical matter, it is my psychiatric/neuropsychiatric opinion—held with a degree of reasonable medical probability—that as of the time of my attempted interview/examination of Mr. Princely, his inferrable mental state and psychiatric/neuropsychiatric condition *would* support a legal/court determination that he is *not* presently and is *not* likely to become (for the reasonably foreseeable future) competent to stand trial (CST), because of his present and anticipated future (for the reasonably foreseeable future) lack of "ability to participate with counsel [you] in an adequate presentation of his defense."

While I cannot at this point offer a clinical diagnostic impression (psychiatric/neuropsychiatric) about Mr. Princely; while I am aware of his lack of a psychiatric history or of psychiatric treatment; and while I am aware (from our discussions) that Mr. Princely has in the past spoken with you and cooperated with you, as a practical present (and foreseeable future) clinical matter, Mr. Princely's withdrawn, uninvolved, and uncooperative behaviors prevent him from demonstrating the "ability to participate with counsel in an adequate presentation of his defense."

From a clinical perspective, the differential diagnosis (i.e., the factors, diagnoses, clinical conditions, or other such issues that might be the cause of an individual's clinical presentation) of Mr. Princely's present clinical presentation includes malingering, as well as psychotic or prepsychotic conditions.

At this time, this cause is not known to me, but again, as a practical matter, Mr. Princely's clinical presentation—in my professional psychiatric/neuropsychiatric opinion—prevents him from having the present "Ability to participate with counsel in an adequate presentation of his defense."

Last, Dr. Liebman wrote the customary disclaimers, distinguishing his forensic report from a purely clinical one.

The referenced individual was examined with reference to specific circumstances emanating from the incident in question, in accordance with the restrictive rules concerning an independent medical examination. It is, therefore, understood that no treatment was given or suggested, and that no doctor/patient relationship exists.

I aver that the information contained in this document was prepared by the undersigned and is the work of the undersigned. It is true to the best of my knowledge and information, and has not been modified by anyone other than the undersigned.

Please advise me if you have questions about this evaluation and report, or if you anticipate requiring additional services from me in connection with this matter.

Thank you very much.

Sincerely,

Klaus Liebman, MD, MS

Diplomate, American Board of Psychiatry and Neurology (P)

Certified, American Society of Addiction Medicine

Case Analysis and Overview

In this matter, Mr. Princely had a long-standing history of psychiatric disorder, although his lengthy history of criminal behaviors and adjudications and custodial sentences lent considerable validity to an overlay of malingering and feigned psychotic-level mental illness.

Ultimately, the professional mental health consultant/evaluator could not arrive at a professional opinion—held with a degree of reasonable medical probability—about inferences about Mr. Princely's underlying mental state and psychiatric/neuropsychiatric/addiction medicine condition with respect to the question of his being considered competent to stand trial. This evaluator returned approximately two weeks later for another attempt at an evaluation, with the same result as the first time.

Procedurally, owing to Mr. Princely's lengthy (extended term) state prison incarceration for a number of offenses, his prison term sentence at the point that the mental health consultant/evaluator attempted to interview/examine him was for another 25 years.

From the perspective of the pointers discussed in Chapter 1, owing to the time pressures imposed on all involved in this case by the court, the total time from Dr. Liebman's retention by the court to the time of his evaluation and report was only two weeks. This underscores the need, especially in court-appointed evaluations in our experience, for quick response time and active communication with all involved in a case, especially trial court judges.

Approximately two months after that second attempt, Mr. Princely was court-ordered to be transferred to the state hospital for the criminally insane (a state psychiatric facility that evaluates and treats inmates in correctional settings who require a more intense level of treatment than the correctional institutions themselves; these institutions have a variety of names, including "hospitals for the criminally insane," "forensic centers," and others). At that facility, Mr. Princely initially refused to accept psychotropic medication (including antipsychotic medication). However, after an incident of violence against a hospital professional staff member by Mr. Princely, he was force-medicated with antipsychotic medication, which continued over a period of several months. This pharmacotherapy did not produce a clinically significant improvement; however, it did result in a lower level of acting-out and violence and dangerousness on Mr. Princely's part.

The issue of Mr. Princely's CST status was never resolved, as a practical matter, and his escape charges were also never resolved.

State v. William Kreech

Case Overview: Malingering

The issue in this case was to determine whether the defendant, William Kreech, who was in prison on a sex offense conviction, was competent to stand trial (CST) on another charge alleged to have been committed while incarcerated. The Honorable Stephen A. Douglas, JSC (Judge of the Superior Court), retained the services of a psychiatrist, Hans Poulter, MD, relevant to that determination. Dr. Poulter's report follows.

The Report

> One of the bread-and-butter forensic issues frequently evaluated by mental health professionals is that of a defendant's competency to stand trial. As with many other areas in forensic mental health evaluations, however, a good deal of subjectivity may be encountered in interpreting an evaluee's competency status, putting the evaluator in a position to be skeptical about the motives for the evaluee's possibly feigning psychiatric symptomatology, and requiring that the evaluator consider malingering in the differential diagnosis of the evaluee's clinical presentation. As with the previous report *(State v. Theodore Princely)*, the writer of this report states the nature and scope of the report in a direct, concise, and straightforward way, even if the issues to be discussed are not straightforward in themselves.

Following up on our telephone discussion and correspondence about the above-referenced matter, I am writing you this report of my psychiatric/neuro-psychiatric evaluation of Mr. William Kreech in connection with this matter.

This report is provided at your request, and is intended to give you my psychiatric/neuropsychiatric opinion—held with a degree of reasonable medical probability—about Mr. Kreech's mental state and psychiatric/neuropsychiatric condition and mental state with regard to the legal/forensic psychiatric issue of his present competency to stand trial (CST), in connection with an incident that had allegedly occurred at Valley Prison (VP). During that incident, Mr. Kreech had allegedly set his spare clothing in his cell on fire on two occasions, eventually resulting in a plea agreement for an additional four years of incarceration in state prison. As I understand from our initial telephone discussion about this matter on January 6, XXXX, Mr. Kreech is presently serving a state prison sentence for a sex offense, and had been eligible for parole in XXXX, prior to the alleged fire-setting incidents.

Although information about Mr. Kreech's relatively recent history at VP is unclear, he told your court, through the VP ombudsman (advocacy) program, that he was taking medications prescribed by a professional health care staff member at VP. He also told the ombudsman that the staff at that facility had evaluated him for his CST status in connection with that incident. He was reportedly determined by that staff to be CST, although that report is from Mr. Kreech, and to my knowledge and understanding, documentation of any such evaluations has not yet been made available for review.

Because of the problematic nature of Mr. Kreech's competency, the Superior Court Judge took it upon himself to arrange for a court-appointed mental health evaluator to be certain that a mental and objective evaluation would be done so that an independent and objective professional would do this potentially difficult evaluation. Usually defense counsel arranges for competency evaluations, and the State (prosecution) will retain another evaluator for a second opinion in potentially complicated cases.

In any event, as you described in the "Reason for Use of Expert and Theory or Admissibility" section of the "Expert Witness Request Form" in this matter, "Client is in State Prison. He is setting fires in the prison and is either unwilling or is unable to assist counsel. Competency and possible NGI determination" were requested.

Records and materials reviewed for this particular evaluation were very limited, primarily because the concern of the court (to be addressed by the forensic evaluator) was focused only on Mr. Kreech's present and anticipated future mental state and psychiatric/neuropsychiatric condition with regard to his competency to stand trial status. The court order for this evaluation is discussed next in this report.

With this introductory background and information, I note that to date, medical records and materials from VP, and more recently from South State Prison (SSP), to which facility Mr. Kreech has been transferred, as described below are not available for my review in this evaluation. In the event that situation changes, and in the event that such information significantly changes my professional opinions in this matter, I anticipate providing you with a supplemental report incorporating such information, if indicated and requested, at a future date. For the present, however, I reiterate that this evaluation and report are clinically oriented and based on my interview/examination of Mr. Kreech at the Bonner County Jail (BCJ), to which facility Mr. Kreech had been transferred temporarily for procedural purposes pertaining to this matter.

Finally, by way of background and history, I note that my interview/examination of Mr. Kreech occurred on September 10, XXXX. This was the third of three attempts to interview/examine Mr. Kreech: The first was scheduled for May 11, XXXX, and would have occurred at VP, but Mr. Kreech had been transferred by that time to SSP without notice to you. My second effort to interview/examine Mr. Kreech was on August 23, XXXX, at the BCJ; however, when I arrived at that facility, I was advised by staff that the additional security necessary to support that interview/examination was not available. I returned on September 10, XXXX, and was able to conduct an interview/examination of Mr. Kreech. That interview/examination, however, was not altogether satisfactory, because of Mr. Kreech's lack of cooperation.

In terms of the parameters of the evaluation, they are set forth in the following excerpts from the applicable court order, authored by The Honorable John Jefferson, JSC:

What follows is a lengthy excerpt from Judge Douglas's court order for the competency evaluation, reiterating and emphasizing the specific points to be addressed in the evaluation.

Pursuant to (applicable statute), defendant is to be examined, by Dr. Hans Poulter, at Valley Prison, on May 11, XXXX, from 1:30 P.M. until examination is completed, in order to determine whether hospitalization is clinically necessary to perform an examination for fitness to proceed. As the defendant is an inmate in Valley Prison, the prison staff shall permit such examination at the jail or prison and shall provide access to relevant medical psychiatrist or psychological reports and records in their possession. . . . If Dr. Hans Poulter determines that hospitalization is unnecessary to perform an examination for fitness to proceed, the qualified psychiatrist or licensed psychologist shall perform the examination at the jail or prison. . . . If the qualified psychiatrist or licensed psychologist determines that hospitalization is necessary to perform an examination for fitness to proceed, then the defendant shall be committed to the custody of the Commissioner of Human Services for placement for that purpose for a period not exceeding thirty (30) days . . . the finding of the qualified psychiatrist or licensed psychologist conducting the examination shall be submitted in a written report to this court and shall include:

(a) A description of the nature of the examination;
(b) A diagnosis of the mental condition of the defendant;
(c) An opinion as to the defendant's capacity to understand the proceeding against him and to assist in his own defense;
(d) An opinion as to the defendant's present competence to proceed to trial;
(e) An opinion as to whether defendant's mental condition is such that he poses a present danger either to himself, to others, or to property upon his release into the general community.

Dr. Poulter next writes a final paragraph summarizing the events that led to the present evaluation and describing its nature and scope.

As mentioned above, it is my understanding that as a result of Mr. Kreech's having reportedly set his spare clothing on fire twice in the relatively recent past "I do not know specific dates" (his words), he has been "twice charged with Arson in the second degree" (excerpted from Judge Jefferson's "Order for a Psychiatric or Psychological Examination of Defendant's Fitness to Proceed and Defendant's Dangerousness to Self, Others, or Property as a Result of Mental Illness"). By virtue of Mr. Kreech's presentation, past psychiatric history, apparently prescribed psychotropic medications, this present psychiatric/neuropsychiatric evaluation was ordered, in anticipation of further recommendations, if indicated, for further efforts (i.e., psychiatric hospitalization) to assess Mr. Kreech's mental state/psychiatric/neuropsychiatric condition in the context of his CST status.

Mr. Kreech's history is mentioned briefly in this report, which next focuses on interview/examination findings, impressions, and the opinions of the evaluator. Those observations, findings, impressions, and opinions—as in the previous report—were presented succinctly in order to enhance communications with the court (an important pointer for forensic mental health experts).

On interview/examination in interview room on the first floor of the BCJ on September 10, XXXX, Mr. Kreech presented as a tall, well-developed, well-nourished Caucasian male who was dressed in the dark green short-sleeved BCJ outfit and wore hiking boots.

I introduced myself to him, ascertained his understanding of the purpose and scope of the interview/examination, and advised him of the likelihood nonconfidential nature of the evaluation. He told me this was acceptable to him. We then proceeded with the interview/examination.

Throughout the interview/examination, Mr. Kreech did not maintain eye contact, periodically stared into space, and commented that he was hearing voices.

Initially, I asked Mr. Kreech what his understanding was of who I was and why he was in the BCJ and he replied responsively but stating, "I don't know. Where are you? Where are all of us? Where are we all going?" I continued by attempting to introduce myself to Mr. Kreech and to discuss the nature and purpose of this interview/examination and evaluation with him. I specifically told him about my understanding about having set his mattresses at Valley Prison on fire and about the resulting institutional infraction charges against him. I then asked him what he would tell me about having burned his mattresses. He said that, "I wanted to lay on the mattress, to send myself to Hell. To burn myself to Hell . . . ." In response to my question about how many times he burned his mattress, Mr. Kreech replied "six"; and in response to my question about where he burned his mattresses, he said he did not know, but "my friend Baby M. told me to." I also asked him about medications that were being given to him through the Medical Department of BCJ (at that time) and SSP since his transfer there. He told me, "A lot, I don't know what they are." I repeated the question, obtaining another "I don't know" response. At that point anticipating no further cooperation with Mr. Kreech in terms of his background, history, the history of the mattress burning incidents, and so forth, I next reviewed the several elements of CST, according to applicable statutory law, as I understand that law. Mr. Kreech's responses were as follows:

- Mr. Kreech's *Charges* according to him, are "I don't know."
- In terms of *Orientation* questions having to do with time, person, place, and circumstances of reasons for this interview/examination, he told me that he thought he was "in prison here, I'm not too sure."
- A *Court of Law,* according to Mr. Kreech is a "bunch of pigs, play in the mud, drinking coffee, eating straw."
- A *Judge,* according to Mr. Kreech is a "a devil. I heard some things about him. The devil. Anytime you want, come and join him with a razor."
- A *Jury,* according to Mr. Kreech, is: "He's a demon. Six of them."
- A *Prosecuting Attorney,* according to Mr. Kreech, is "the devil's advocate, his son, the devil."
- A *Defense Counsel,* according to Mr. Kreech, is "the hot water that burns, burns to go to hell, shake the devil's hand in advance."
- Mr. Kreech's understanding of the *Plea Bargaining/Negotiation* process is: "I don't know, I don't know, all I know is death and suicide. Anything to do with blood."
- Whether or not an individual may be *Compelled to Testify About Him/ Herself,* according to Mr. Kreech, is "no." When I asked him why this was, he replied, "I don't know."
- Finally, Mr. Kreech's opinion about his present *Ability to Participate With Counsel in an Adequate Presentation of His Defense* is: "I don't know."

Mr. Kreech's clinical presentation has already been discussed. He was not cooperative with me throughout the interview/examination, and the inconsistency

> Dr. Poulter next summarized his findings in the final two paragraphs of this section of his report.

between his understanding the nature of the interview/examination and some of my questions (particularly about his CST status) indicated overt faking, and efforts to simulate psychosis in unsophisticated ways on Mr. Kreech's part (e.g., his awareness of my question of what a jury is—"He's a demon"—was in my opinion a clumsy attempt on Mr. Kreech's part to appear psychotic).

Otherwise, Mr. Kreech's appearance and presentation were as described above. Throughout this interview/examination, as mentioned above, he did not maintain eye contact, stared off into space, and unconvincingly told me that he was responding to voices. "I don't know, just voices."

> The "Clinical Diagnostic Impressions" and the "Summary and Opinions" sections of this report were merged together and not presented as separate sections of the report. However, the straightforward opinions of the evaluator, as expressed toward the end of the report, were that "Mr. William Kreech's clinical presentation as of the time of my interview/examination of him was consistent with malingering psychosis on his part on the one hand, and that on the other, he does have the capacity to understand the proceeding against him and assist in his own defense."

From a diagnostic perspective, while I recognize that Mr. Kreech may—independent of his malingering—have a psychiatric history and a legitimate psychiatric diagnosis, without cooperation on his part; without other medical records and materials to review (if any exist) pertaining to him historically or presently (i.e., medical records and materials from the Medical Department at the SSP and BCJ); and without independent knowledge or information on my part about Mr. Kreech's psychiatric background and history (if any), the only diagnostic formulation that I can reach presently in terms of this evaluation is that Mr. Kreech is malingering to appear psychotic, likely for purposes of secondary gain (e.g., to be discharged from prison and be transferred to Bayway Mental Hospital), by virtue of his unsophisticated and, in my view, ineffective simulation of psychosis.

In terms of the issue (described in the above court order) of Mr. Kreech's transfer to the Commissioner of Human Services for an extended period of inpatient forensic psychiatric evaluation concerning Mr. Kreech's CST status, while such an additional period of observation would be useful from a clinical perspective to clarify Mr. Kreech's mental state and psychiatric/neuropsychiatric/addiction medicine (if applicable) condition and diagnosis, such an extended period of evaluation is not necessary, in my professional opinion, to address the issue of Mr. Kreech's present (and anticipated future) CST status, according to applicable statutory, as I understand that law.

> Toward the end of his report, Dr. Poulter again requested copies of whatever additional records and materials might be available for review in anticipation of a possible follow-up, supplemental report. Such a request—a disclaimer, in effect, indicating the potential change of impressions and opinions that any additional records could bring about—should routinely be made for any expert report. Additional records and materials could almost always be obtained, and the potential effect they might have on an expert's opinion simply cannot be known in advance of reviewing such records.

In this last regard, I do request copies of criminal/discovery records and materials and medical/psychiatric records and materials that are probably available in Mr. Kreech's files, for the reasons described above. In the event that the information learned from these additional records and materials significantly change my professional psychiatric/neuropsychiatric opinion—held with a degree of reasonable medical probability—in this matter, I anticipate providing you with a supplemental report incorporating information learned from these additional sources at a future date, if indicated and requested.

However, for present purposes, it is my psychiatric/neuropsychiatric opinion—held with a degree of reasonable medical probability—that Mr. William Kreech's clinical presentation as of the time of my interview/examination of him was consistent with malingering psychosis on his part on the one hand; and on the other, that he does have the "capacity to understand the proceeding against him and to assist in his own defense." He has present competence to proceed to trial if he chooses to do so, and by virtue of his present malingering and uncertain psychiatric/neuropsychiatric condition and presentation in the face of having recently reportedly setting his clothing in his VP cell on fire twice, he does pose a present danger either to himself, to other persons, and to property as of the time of my interview/examination of him and for the reasonably foreseeable future after that.

> Last, Dr. Poulter wrote the customary disclaimers, distinguishing his forensic report from a purely clinical one.

The referenced individual was examined with reference to specific circumstances emanating from the incident in question, in accordance with the restrictive rules concerning an independent medical examination. It is, therefore, understood that no treatment was given or suggested, and that no doctor/patient relationship exists.

I aver that the information contained in this document was prepared by the undersigned and is the work of the undersigned. It is true to the best of my knowledge and information, and has not been modified by anyone other than the undersigned.

Please keep me informed about whether or not criminal/discovery and medical/psychiatric records and materials will be made available to me (as indicated in the above-mentioned court order pertaining to this evaluation) for this matter.

In the meantime please do not hesitate to contact me if you have questions about this present evaluation and report, or if you anticipate requiring additional services from me in connection with this matter.

Thank you very much.

Sincerely,

Hans Poulter, MD, MS

Diplomate, American Board of Psychiatry and Neurology (P)

Certified, American Society of Addiction Medicine

Case Analysis and Outcome

In forensic mental health practice, unlike clinical practice, an evaluating practitioner must maintain skepticism about the motivations and truthfulness of the history and clinical presentation given by evaluees. In that sense, malingering must always be considered in the *differential diagnosis* (the list of conditions that could cause a given clinical presentation or pattern of symptoms potentially relevant to forensic mental health concern at issue) of the individual being evaluated. In this case, the combination of Mr. Kreech's lack of any known psychotic-level psychiatric history along with his nonsensical and stereotyped clinical presentation (as if imitating a crazy person) led to the examiner's opinion that inferences about Mr. Kreech's underlying mental state and psychiatric/neuropsychiatric/addiction medicine condition as of the time of his evaluation *do* support Mr. Kreech's malingering psychosis on the one hand, but do not support his being considered not CST.

In addition, in this case, owing to the dangerous and violent way Mr. Kreech had behaved prior to and at the time of the evaluation, the mental health evaluator offered the opinion that Mr. Kreech is likely to act out again in a dangerous way in the reasonably foreseeable future, especially if it serves his purposes to do so. This opinion also supported Mr. Kreech's having been malingering during the time surrounding the interview/examination.

In this particular case, about three months after Dr. Poulter's initial evaluation, Mr. Kreech set another mattress on fire. He was investigated by authorities, "confessed" (his word) that he had set the previous fires "to try to look crazy and get sent to a hospital" (his words). When he finally realized that that tactic would not be effective, he "gave up, I confess . . . I won't do it again." A follow-up and supplemental report by Dr. Poulter was not necessary.

State v. Adolph Taylor

Case Overview: Child (Sexual) Abuse

The defendant in this matter, Adolph Taylor, was charged with the multiple counts of sexual assault involving his daughter both when she was a child and a young adult. Defense counsel, Paul Guidry, Esquire, requested an evaluation of the defendant to determine if there was a possible criminal responsibility-reducing defense. Counsel retained Curtis Bollinger, MD, MPH, for a relevant evaluation. Dr. Bollinger's report follows.

The Report

> This is a straightforward evaluation. It focuses on the classical forensic psychiatric question of the applicability of a criminal responsibility-reducing (or eliminating, in the case of the "Legal Insanity") psychiatric defense for alleged criminal acts, and follows the full clinically based report format described in Chapter 1. By way of introduction, the report first discusses the nature, scope, issues addressed, and objectives of the report, and then lists and summarizes the sources of information (including summaries of records reviewed) for the evaluation.

Following up on our telephone discussions and correspondence about the above-referenced matter, and based on the sources of information given below, I am writing you this report of my psychiatric/neuropsychiatric/addiction medicine evaluation of Mr. Adolph Taylor in connection with this matter.

As you and I discussed shortly after my interview/examination of Mr. Taylor at the Butler County Prison (BCP) on August 10, XXXX, my psychiatric/neuropsychiatric/addiction medicine opinion about inferences about Mr. Taylor's mental state and psychiatric/neuropsychiatric/addiction medicine condition during the period of time surrounding his alleged sexual offenses against his daughter, Mabel Taylor, in this matter, would *not* support a criminal responsibility-reducing "traditional" (my word) psychiatric defense, such as "Legal Insanity," "Diminished Capacity," and/or "Intoxication."

> Although issues of substance abuse did not specifically pertain to Mr. Taylor's mental state or clinical condition in connection with his alleged offenses in this matter, the scope of Dr. Bollinger's evaluation included inquiry into possible substance abuse issues in this matter. Therefore, the designation "psychiatric/neuropsychiatric/addiction medicine" is used throughout this report.

Similarly, since my psychiatric/neuropsychiatric/addiction medicine opinion in this matter would also not support a legal/court determination that Mr. Taylor was *not* able to have "knowingly, intelligently, and voluntarily" waived his constitutional rights at the time of his interrogation in this matter, I will not structure this report as a usual forensic psychiatric/neuropsychiatric/addiction medicine evaluation concerning Mr. Taylor's mental states and psychiatric/neuropsychiatric conditions during those several periods of time.

Rather, after initially listing and discussing the records and materials that I reviewed in connection with this evaluation and report, I will present and discuss Mr. Taylor's background and history leading up to the period of time of his alleged sexual assaults against his daughter; will present and discuss those offenses from the perspectives of the discovery records and materials as well as from his own perspectives, and their investigation and aftermath; will present and discuss my psychiatric/neuropsychiatric observations and findings concerning Mr. Taylor; will present and discuss my clinical diagnostic impressions of Mr. Taylor; and will conclude this report (in the "Summary and Opinions" section of the report) with a clinically based and clinically oriented discussion of Mr. Taylor's psychiatric/neuropsychiatric condition and situation, with recommendations for his disposition—again, from a clinical psychiatric/neuropsychiatric perspective—in the context of the above-referenced matter, to the extent that these recommendations may be feasible in this matter.

After giving an overview of the scope and structure of the report, Dr. Bollinger next presents and summarizes the bases of the report.

The sources of information on which this evaluation and report are based are as follows:

1. My review of copies of criminal/legal/discovery records and materials provided to me by your office in connection with this matter, as follows (for reasons discussed below, no medical or clinical records or materials existed, for review in this matter).

Criminal/legal discovery records and materials pertaining to sexual assault incidents between July 18 and July 26, XXXX, in which Mr. Adolph Taylor allegedly "did engage in sexual intercourse with Mabel Taylor, by forcible compulsion . . . without her consent . . . did have indecent contact with another person and/or did cause another person to have indecent contact with him, namely, Mabel Taylor . . . [and] . . . did knowingly have sexual intercourse with another, Mabel Taylor, a daughter of whole blood, or without regard to legitimacy or relationship of parent and child by adoption . . . " (language excerpted, in part, from the "Police Criminal Complaint" in this matter).

In the "Affidavit of Probable Cause," the affiant (criminal investigator Porter Vance of the City of Middleville Police Department) wrote the following, by way of background and history to these offenses:

"On July 26, XXXX, the victim Mabel Taylor of 18 Wimberly Road, Middleville, Butler County reported to the Middleville Police Department, she has been being sexually assaulted by her biological father, the DEFENDANT, Adolph Taylor. She can recall the DEFENDANT touching her in a non-appropriate manner since she was been six years old. She stated he began having intercourse with her since she was approximately 10 years old. Intercourse would occur approximately once every two weeks since then.

"On July 18, XXXX at approximately 0800 hours, the DEFENDANT told her to go into his bathroom at 18 Wimberly Road, Middleville, Butler County because he wanted to have sexual intercourse. Sexual intercourse again occurred on July 20, XXXX, again in his bedroom, which is where it always occurred . . . the victim stated the DEFENDANT would repeatedly threaten to physically harm her, her cat, or kick the cat out of the house if she would tell anyone or fail to comply.

"The DEFENDANT has in the past, to include May of XXXX, physically grabbed her by the arm and forced her to have intercourse with him. The victim did have a bruise on her back which was reportedly from being struck by the DEFENDANT . . . the Affiant and Detective Brue served a Search Warrant on the residence at 18 Wimberly Road on July 26, XXXX.

"Detective Brue advised the DEFENDANT of the Probable Cause for the Search Warrant at which the DEFENDANT admitted to having sexual intercourse with his biological daughter on July 25, XXXX.

"The DEFENDANT was then advised of his *Miranda* Warnings and further admitted to having sexual intercourse with the victim, his biological daughter once a week for the past four years. This would include twice having anal intercourse. The DEFENDANT admitted he knew this was wrong to do this to the victim . . . ."

Additional criminal/legal discovery records and materials, Supplementary Police Reports, and other such records were contained in this collection.

The Affidavit of Probable Cause for the search warrant, in which Investigator Vance was the affiant, described the following:

> "On July 21, XXXX, the victim, Mabel Taylor reported to the Middleville Police Department that she had been raped by her father, Adolph Taylor, DOB: 1-14-XXXX on 02-XX-XXXX at 1242 B Lebanon Street, Middleville, Butler County.
> "The victim stated Adolph Taylor used threats and intimidation to force her to comply with his demands. At approximately 0800 hours, Adolph Taylor instructed her to go into his bedroom, he removed her pajama pants and panties and had sexual intercourse with her.
> "Prior to ejaculating, he removed his penis from her vagina and ejaculated on a multi-colored striped bath towel. To the best of the victim's knowledge, Adolph Taylor did not wash the bedding in his bedroom and possibly the bath towel."

Finally, also included in this collection of discovery records and materials was the handwritten statement of Adolph Taylor, transcribed by Detective Brue, dated July 26, XXXX (10:40 P.M.) and taken at Mr. Taylor's home and at the Middleville Police Department's Headquarters.

At the beginning of this statement was Mr. Taylor's signed *Miranda* rights waiver, with the specific "Y" ("Yes") designations for each of the six points in this document initialed by the detective (according to Mr. Taylor's recollection; based on Mr. Taylor's cognitive limitations, to be discussed in further detail below, it is likely that the detective read the *Miranda* items to Mr. Taylor, and that the detective assigned "Y" to indicate Mr. Taylor's understanding and agreement).

For further information and details contained in these several records and materials, the reader is referred to them;

> Mr. Taylor had no significant medical or clinical records or materials provided for review in this matter. His own history is discussed later in the report, and is noteworthy for long-standing cognition impairment. He related an orthopedic and medical history as well, without records, materials, or other documentation to confirm or refute his own reported history.

2. My psychiatric/neuropsychiatric interview/examination of Mr. Adolph Taylor in an interview room at the Butler County Prison (BCP), which interview/examination included the administration and subsequent scoring and interpretation of two standardized cognitive screening tests (the Mini-Mental State Examination, or MMSE, and the Cognitive Capacity Screening Examination, or the CCSE) and a nonstandardized "Past Medical History" questionnaire (which, owing to Mr. Taylor's cognitive limitations, described in further detail below, I completed after asking him questions about his past medical history); and

3. My knowledge, background, training, and experience in psychiatry and neuropsychiatry, addiction medicine, and forensic psychiatry, and—for present purposes, in particular—my work and experience over the years with individuals with various types of organic brain syndrome, both acquired (such as individuals with closed head injuries, and other types of traumatic brain injury) and from birth (individuals with various developmental disabilities, dyslexia, ADHD, mental retardation, and so forth).

> Continuing the report, the "History" section presents the background and history of the alleged perpetrator and the offense at issue, especially discussing how and how long he had engaged in the several offenses at issue.

History

Mr. Adolph Taylor is a 60-year-old (DOB: January 14, XXXX) widowed Caucasian male. His deceased wife, Genevieve Hicks Taylor, died in July of XXXX at the age of 47. Ms. Taylor worked in food preparation at a local university, and was limited cognitively and intellectually herself, having stopped school when she was in the sixth grade and having been placed in a group home when she was 16 years old. The couple married in August of XXXX, by Mr. Taylor's recollection. Mr. Taylor has lived in the upstairs apartment at 18 Wimberly Road in Middleville for 27 years (i.e., up to the time of his arrest and incarceration for the above-mentioned charges). He retired as a stock boy from a local hardware store after 14 years of that work.

Mr. Taylor described that he is presently on SSI through the Butler County Social Services Department, and that he "saw a psychiatrist twice" for evaluation for his SSI (no records or materials about these reported consultations are available for review).

Mr. Taylor and his wife have a daughter, Mabel Mary Taylor (DOB: October 29, XXXX), who herself is handicapped and on SSI by virtue of a seizure disorder and developmental disability.

Mr. Taylor himself is in the middle range of five siblings (three are currently living), three males and two females. His siblings range from 56 years old (a single brother, Hugo, a plumber by training and occupation, currently incarcerated for 10 years for sex offenses, and presently "dying of internal bleeding") to 62 years old (a sister, Wilma Taylor, who is a pensioner on the basis of her blindness).

In addition, Mr. Taylor had a single older brother, Lawrence Taylor, who died in a motor vehicle accident in July of XXXX at the age of 52; and a younger sister, Ethel Salinger, the mother of two sons and two daughters in their 20s, who died of cancer at the age of 50 in XXXX leaving behind a husband who was killed in XXXX in a robbery incident in Illinois.

Mr. Taylor's father, Jerry Taylor, died at the age of 64 of causes unknown to Mr. Taylor, and his mother, Belle Taylor, died at the age of 89, with Alzheimer's disease.

> **Dr. Bollinger also discussed the victim's mother's background and history to complete the clinical picture of the nuclear family.**

For present purposes, I also note Mr. Taylor's account of his deceased wife's family history: Ms. Taylor was one of six siblings (three males and three females), of whom five are still living. According to Mr. Taylor, in addition to his deceased wife's developmental disability/mental retardation, two other siblings—a brother, Paul, now 45 years old, and a sister, Beth, now 67 years old—are also both reportedly cognitively limited and possibly developmentally disabled/mentally retarded (Mr. Taylor did not know the history of his deceased wife's parents in this area).

Mr. Taylor's deceased wife's divorced 62-year-old brother, Mr. John Hicks, is one of the uncles to whom Mr. Taylor referred when he gave his statement of his having had sex with his daughter "because her uncles had." Although not clear to me (Mr. Taylor's demeanor, presentation, and clinical psychiatric/neuropsychiatric condition and status will be discussed in further detail below), the other uncle was possibly Mr. Charles Bell, now 58 years old, and also possibly developmentally disabled/mentally retarded.

Mr. Taylor commented in that context that "David Feist and I are the only ones who got into trouble" for alleged sexual offenses against Mabel Taylor; he also told me that his brother-in-law is also incarcerated for those charges at the BCP.

To the best of Mr. Taylor's knowledge, his *Family History* of several chronic conditions includes cardiovascular disorders (his father, who died of a myocardial infarction and had a "mixed-up heart—skipped beats," and his mother who had a cerebrovascular accident [a "stroke"], a myocardial infarction, and who died with Alzheimer's disease, as noted above); neoplastic (cancer) diseases (his two sisters, one of whom died of possible bone cancer); neurologic disorders (his mother, with Alzheimer's disease); and psychiatric/neuropsychiatric disorders (several family members, as described above, with likely developmental disabilities/mental retardation).

Mr. Taylor denied any known family history of pulmonary disorders; metabolic/endocrine disorders; gastrointestinal/hepatitis disorders; infectious diseases (including STDs and HIV disease); and chemical dependency disorders.

> The report next describes Mr. Taylor's personal, past, and developmental history as a straightforward account of clinical history. The report began with developmental issues, as relevant to Mr. Taylor's long-standing history of developmental disability and cognitive impairment.

By way of his own background and history, Mr. Taylor commented that he did not know about whether his mother's pregnancy with him was planned or wanted, and similarly did not know about his mother's pregnancy or labor and delivery of him, or whether she drank alcohol, used substances of abuse, or had any gynecologic problems (such as eclampsia, hypertension, and so forth) during her pregnancy with him. He also did not know his birth weight, or whether there was any question in his parents' health care providers' or school authorities' minds about developmental delays, disabilities, congenital mental retardation, or other such impairments or limitations for Mr. Taylor, and so forth.

> The possible contribution of psychiatric/neuropsychiatric/addiction medicine developmental factors to Mr. Taylor's subsequent life were not known and not documented through medical, clinical, or related records or materials. Only Mr. Taylor's limited recollection of his history—unreliable at best—gave this information.

Mr. Taylor's family was living in Harleyville at the time of his birth, and his father worked at the local cemetery, by his recollection, "cutting grass and digging graves."

Mr. Taylor commented that he had no specific memories from the time that he was born until the time that he started kindergarten (at 5 years of age), although he did tell me in response to my specific question that there was no history of childhood or later abuse of him by his family or by others, physical, emotional, or sexual.

From kindergarten through the fifth grade, Mr. Taylor attended the Brookwood Elementary School, having been in special education classes throughout, having felt discouraged but "resigned to it," and having been aware that "my report card wasn't good—I couldn't read good."

When Mr. Taylor was in the sixth, seventh, and eighth grades, his family relocated to Proctor, where they lived in what Mr. Taylor described as a rural setting: "A home with an outhouse, we didn't build a bathroom." The family subsequently relocated back to Harleyville.

Mr. Taylor then attended Grayson High School, in grades 9 through 12. He graduated in XXXX at the age of 21, having repeated three grades over the years (he did not remember which ones, during my interview/examination).

> Although not available for review in this case, school and vocational records can be very useful in forensic mental health evaluations of developmentally disabled individuals in civil or criminal matters. Child Study Team records, when applicable and available, can be particularly helpful in describing a (former) student's clinical background and condition as of the time of the multidisciplinary evaluation.

Throughout these years, Mr. Taylor lived with his family until he married in XXXX. His father died, as noted above, in XXXX, and Mr. Taylor lived with his mother for the following 11 years.

Mr. Taylor met his wife, Genevieve Hicks, at a training center for cognitively impaired individuals, and married her approximately one month later. Mr. Taylor described that his wife "wanted to get out of the group home." The couple moved into "projects—she was pregnant—Mabel Mary was born in October, XXXX."

Mr. Taylor described both his wife and his daughter as "slow" (cognitively). For example, his wife "worked at food preparation at the training center for two years, then was fired and didn't go back."

Shortly after his daughter's birth, Mabel was "taken away from us . . . her right leg and shoulder were broken . . . child abuse . . . taken away at one month into foster placement until—two-and-one-half years old. With records about her low calcium, we got her back. My wife was angry, had fits, was abusive . . . screamer."

Despite their early problems with their baby daughter, Mr. Taylor described the first 11 years of their marriage as "good years, good health, steady, stable, I was working." From XXXX to XXXX, Mr. Taylor described "good years" as well, but "Genevieve's cancer started in XXXX. She suffered two-and-one-half years with that."

Concerning Mr. Taylor's account of his history of sexual activities with his daughter, he told me that he "first had sex with Mabel" when she was 16 years old. "My wife was sick, not having sex with me. I turned to Mabel. *I knew it was wrong, but I did it* [emphasis added: See below]. I asked if it was all right, and she pulled her shade in her room down and pulled down her pants and went into

> At this point in the report, after setting out Mr. Taylor's background and history leading to the alleged child abuse offenses in question, Dr. Bollinger described Mr. Taylor's account of those offenses.

my room and lay down on my bed and then we had sex. My wife was downstairs while this happened. She never said anything, but she told me about Johnny [or John Hicks, Mabel's uncle on her mother's side] after one year. My wife didn't believe my daughter about Johnny's having sex with her. It happened just that one time, oral sex. Mabel told me that."

Mr. Taylor commented that he had sex with his daughter approximately twice a month "until I was caught."

Dr. Bollinger concluded this "History" section with Mr. Taylor's brief account of the circumstances of his arrest for these alleged offenses. This was in substantial agreement with police (discovery) accounts of this matter (above).

Finally, Mr. Taylor's account of his arrest and incarceration was that, "I was at the cemetery putting flowers on my wife's grave, and I went home and put my bike away. I drank beer, and the police came by and arrested me. My daughter was lying. She was sixteen years old and saying I forced her. I never did. I said, 'Is it okay?'"

In the "Mental Status (Psychiatric) Examination" section of the report, the emphasis is on the evaluee's present (i.e., as of the time of the interview/examination) mental status, for evaluating the defendant's competency to stand trial status. Although not a central feature of the evaluation, this assessment is included as a routine matter in order to provide a full and complete evaluation.

Mental Status (Psychiatric) Examination

Mr. Taylor presented in the interview area of the BCP as a tall, heavyset, well-developed, well-nourished white male who was dressed in the short-sleeved brown BCP outfit with an underlying white tee-shirt. He had several days of beard growth, and thick black hair. He wore blue cloth loafers.

I introduced myself to Mr. Taylor, ascertained his understanding of the purpose and scope of the interview/examination, and advised him of the likelihood nonconfidential nature of the evaluation. He told me this was acceptable to him. We then proceeded with the interview/examination.

Throughout the interview/examination, Mr. Taylor appeared tense and anxious, with a fixed smile throughout the process.

Mr. Taylor's demeanor and presentation were those of a cognitively limited and developmentally disabled person overall, with slow, halting speech, limited ability to read (for example, he was only able to read the nonconfidentiality notice very slowly and haltingly, making a number of mistakes, and not understanding that notice without a good deal of discussion and reinforcement on my part).

Mr. Taylor gave the impression of a limited young child, who was working hard to cooperate and participate in this interview/examination.

With the exception of his general level of tenseness and anxiety during this interview/examination, Mr. Taylor did not present with indications of severe affective disorder or symptomatology (such as severe depression, mania, or suicidality). Similarly, he did not present with indications of active thought disorder or psychotic processes or symptomatology (such as hallucinations, delusions, loosening of associations, and so forth).

The predominant way in which Mr. Taylor presented was with confusion, uncertainty about his interactions with me, and otherwise a lack of the subtleties and nuances of this evaluation.

> By this point in this section, Dr. Bollinger has emphasized Mr. Taylor's developmental disability and cognitive impairment. The significance of that is given in the last section ("Summary and Opinions").

Owing to Mr. Taylor's cognitive limitations and impairment, I did not administer the full battery of psychological, chemical dependency, and related tests and inventories that I customarily do. His responses to the two standardized cognitive screening tests (the MMSE and the CCSE) did not indicate gross cognitive impairment, and his responses to the "Past Medical History" questionnaire (which I read to him, because of his limited ability to read, and the responses to which I recorded) were consistent with Mr. Taylor's narrative discussion of his history.

Mr. Taylor noted three medical hospitalizations, two for orthopedic reasons and one for cardiac reasons; denied ever having had a psychiatric problem or chemical dependency problem (including alcohol) requiring treatment; denied any medical illnesses that required treatment for more than two weeks; denied ever having been prescribed psychotropic or nonpsychotropic medications for more than two weeks; described his having been a special education student for most, if not all, of his years of formal education; and also described a long history of manual labor type work (the longest having been as a hardware store stock boy, from XXXX through XXXX; Mr. Taylor told me that he had been trying to get a job since then, but that the "jobs are all filled").

Finally, Mr. Taylor indicated that his present charges are the only criminal charges he has ever faced, and the only criminal activities in which he has allegedly engaged.

> To reiterate: Records and materials to confirm or refute this history reported by Mr. Taylor are not available for the evaluator's review. As a practical matter, that deficiency was not significant for this evaluation, as described below.

In the context of this present evaluation and report, I reviewed with Mr. Taylor the elements of mental competency to stand trial (at present and for the reasonably foreseeable future), according to applicable statutory law, as I understand that law. To my understanding, those elements incorporate the analogous requirements for such competency in the laws (specifically, an understanding of the charges against an individual, and an ability to participate with defense counsel in an adequate presentation of the defendant's case), as follows:

- Mr. Taylor's description of the *Charges* which he is facing are "having relationships with my daughter. Sexual, since she was 16 years old."
- Mr. Taylor's *Orientation* was full (to time, person, place, and circumstances of and reasons for this interview/examination), as determined by his responses to the two standardized cognitive screening tests (the MMSE and the CCSE) as well as by the face-to-face interview/examination.
- Mr. Taylor's understanding of a *Court of Law* was where an individual goes "for a crime that's wrong—get sentencing."
- Mr. Taylor's understanding of a *Jury* was "hear[s] the case and make[s] the ruling, guilty or not guilty."
- Mr. Taylor's response about a *Judge* was an individual to whom a defendant "tell[s] him the truth, and have the case and then give you the ruling, the sentence."
- Mr. Taylor's definition of a *Prosecuting Attorney* was the "attorney for the plaintiff, the state is the plaintiff, to find the defendant guilty."
- Mr. Taylor's understanding of a *Defense Attorney* was the attorney to "defend me, the defendant, less jail time, if he can."
- Mr. Taylor's response to the issue of *Testifying Against Himself* was "I think so." (After discussing this issue further, Mr. Taylor seemed to understand, at least superficially, that this was not the case.)
- Mr. Taylor's explanation of the *Plea Bargaining/Negotiating Process* was that it is intended to "work out charges, how long you get for a sentence, get less sentencing."
- Finally, Mr. Taylor's assessment of his ability to *Cooperate With His Defense Counsel in an Adequate Presentation of His Defense* was "Yes, I can, I can tell what happened and what I think."

Clinical Diagnostic Impressions

In keeping with the current diagnostic nomenclature and format of the *Diagnostic and Statistical Manual of Mental Disorders, Fourth Edition, Text Revision* (2000) of the American Psychiatric Association, clinical diagnostic impressions for Adolph Taylor can be presented as follows:

Axis I (Clinical Disorders):

Cognitive Disorder NOS ("Not Otherwise Specified").
This is discussed in the context of Mr. Taylor's "Borderline Intellectual Functioning," below.

Axis II (Personality Disorders):

Borderline Intellectual Functioning.

Although not formally tested, my clinical impression of Mr. Taylor's cognitive impairment—probably on the basis of genetic and psychosocial deprivation factors—puts him in this range of limited intellectual functioning. While such a range is not *per se* supportive of a "psychiatric defense" (my use of this phrase in this context), it has implications in terms of Mr. Taylor's recommended disposition in this matter, from a clinical psychiatric/neuropsychiatric perspective, as described below.

> This is an important point in terms of the use to which the author's report and opinion may be put, regardless of whether the evaluation is for defense, prosecution, or the court. Not all forensic mental health reports in criminal law are used strictly to support (or not support) a psychiatric defense. Other applications may include sentencing and treatment recommendation purposes, as discussed in Chapter 1.

Axis III (General Medical Conditions):

Mr. Taylor is in generally good medical health presently, without indications of active, acute, chronic, or ongoing medical problems or conditions of clinical significance requiring treatment.

Mr. Taylor's surgical (traumatic) history is as described above.

Axis IV (Psychosocial and Environmental Problems):

Mr. Taylor's main present "Psychosocial and Environmental Problems," in my view at this point, consist of his "Interactions with the legal system/crime," in connection with his present charges and his prospects for further incarceration.

In addition, Mr. Taylor's loss of his wife (in terms of "Problems with primary support group") has been emotionally difficult for him for the past several years. Otherwise, Mr. Taylor appears to have lived a stable, independent, and self-supporting life and lifestyle, even allowing for his cognitive impairment and limitations.

Axis V (Global Assessment of Functioning [GAF]):

A Global Assessment of Functioning (GAF) Scale score for Adolph Taylor of 50–60 signifying moderate-to-serious impairment and symptomatology, in my opinion, applies here.

Summary and Opinions

Mr. Adolph Taylor is a 60-year-old (DOB: January 14, XXXX) widowed, developmentally disabled white male, formerly a manual laborer (most recently, a

Finally, as in all of the forensic reports in this book, the "Summary and Opinions" section pulls together loose ends from other sections of the report; is invariably the section at which the reader begins reading the report to learn an overview of the case and evaluation; and in our experience, is sometimes the only section read by the retaining counsel or the court, unless absolutely necessary (e.g., on the "eve of trial"). It is undoubtedly the most important part of the report, for these reasons. In this particular case, the evaluation was complicated by the evaluee's limited cognitive and intellectual states (and his difficulty accepting that his sexual offenses against his daughter were wrong, notwithstanding his openly acknowledging that they were), and the occurrence of the sexual offenses repeatedly—not simply once or twice, on impulse—over a sustained period of time. This last section of the report addresses that issue head-on, as it should ("would not support a criminal responsibility-reducing psychiatric defense in this matter"). This is another pointer for forensic reports.

stock boy), currently on SSI for his cognitive impairment, as I understand his situation.

Mr. Taylor and his wife had one child, a (now) 24-year-old daughter, Mabel Taylor, herself developmentally disabled.

Mr. Taylor was charged in July of XXXX with repeated sexual assaults on his daughter, Mabel Taylor, as described above and elsewhere in records and materials available for review in this matter. In order to explore forensic psychiatric/neuropsychiatric issues of Mr. Taylor's mental state and psychiatric/neuropsychiatric condition during the periods of time surrounding his allegedly having had sexual intercourse with his daughter, your office arranged for this present psychiatric/neuropsychiatric evaluation of Mr. Taylor for the reasons and via the circumstances described above.

The sources of information on which this evaluation and report are based; Mr. Taylor's background and history; the history of the incident in question and its aftermath; my clinical observations and findings of Mr. Taylor; and my clinical diagnostic impressions are all as described above and elsewhere in records and materials available for review in this matter. That information will not be repeated in this section of this report.

After summarizing the nature, scope, and reasons for this evaluation, Dr. Bollinger next presents his expert forensic opinions.

As a practical matter, and as also noted at the beginning of this present report, inferences that in my professional opinion—held with a degree of reasonable medical probability—can be made about Mr. Taylor's mental state and psychiatric/neuropsychiatric condition during periods of time relevant to this matter (i.e., during the periods of time surrounding the alleged offenses themselves; during the period of time surrounding his "Mirandizing" in this matter; and at present and for the reasonably foreseeable future, in terms of his competency to stand trial status) would not support a criminal responsibility-reducing psychiatric defense in this matter.

Based on the sources of information described above, while Mr. Taylor does show clear cognitive impairment and limitations, he nevertheless in a general sense has sufficient cognitive ability to support a legal/court determination that he was aware of what he was allegedly doing during his reported sexual assaults on his daughter and was aware that what he was reportedly doing was wrong; that he was able to have knowingly, voluntarily, and intelligently waived his Constitutional *(Miranda)* rights when he did, in connection with his statement in this matter; and that he is presently and for the reasonably foreseeable future competent to stand trial, according to applicable state law, as I understand that law.

Therefore, again, I will not discuss Mr. Taylor's clinical psychiatric/neuropsychiatric condition in terms of potential criminal responsibility-reducing psychiatric defenses for him, either for the alleged offenses themselves, or concerning his CST status.

Next, the report shifts to a more clinical orientation, in discussing the author's recommendations for a clinical and therapeutic disposition—and not a strictly custodial one—for this needy and limited defendant.

As noted above in a number of different contexts, Mr. Adolph Taylor is an extremely limited individual cognitively, and a marginal individual in terms of day-to-day activities and level of functioning. He has been able to earn a living and live independently for many years, despite his impairment, and has raised a daughter with his deceased wife (who was also limited), despite his impairment.

In what may be construed as a confused way, Mr. Taylor engaged in inappropriate sexual activities with his daughter for the inappropriate reasons that he described, but which at the time seemed reasonable to him, given his limitations and cognitive impairment.

These comments are not to excuse Mr. Taylor's alleged sexual activities with his daughter, but rather to explain them in the context of an individual with limited cognitive abilities who does not have the level of understanding or sophistication about his unacceptable acts that an individual without his limitations does.

Taking an individual with Mr. Taylor's tenuous and fragile cognitive state, limitations, and impairment into account, from a practical clinical psychiatric/neuropsychiatric perspective, a disposition for him in connection with this matter in a custodial setting would not, in my view, serve toward his clinical improvement or understanding, or rehabilitation. In that sense, such a disposition would be clinically contraindicated.

However, placement of Mr. Taylor in a therapeutic program involving sex offender-specific treatment for developmentally disabled individuals with sexual behavior problems (along the lines of the text materials I sent you on April 15, XXXX) would be strongly clinically indicated as a way of helping Mr. Adolph Taylor address his inappropriate sexual behaviors and thoughts about sexual issues, and as a way of preventing his clinical psychiatric/neuropsychiatric decompensation and deterioration.

Such a therapeutic setting, in my professional opinion, would benefit both Mr. Taylor and his developmentally disabled daughter, the latter of whom must be at least confused and ambivalent about her feelings and wishes toward her father.

Finally, Dr. Bollinger summarizes briefly both his forensic opinions and clinical recommendations in this matter, in a brief concluding paragraph.

In summary, it is my forensic psychiatric/neuropsychiatric opinion—held with a degree of reasonable medical probability—that inferences that may be made about Mr. Adolph Taylor's mental state and psychiatric/neuropsychiatric condition in terms of his mental competency at the times of the offenses in question; at the time of his "Mirandizing" in this matter; and at present and for the reasonably foreseeable future (in the context of his competency to stand trial) would *not* support a legal/court determination for a criminal responsibility-reducing defense in this matter. Nevertheless, from a clinical perspective, it is my psychiatric/neuropsychiatric opinion and recommendation that Mr. Taylor's disposition in this matter be to a therapeutic placement offering sex offender-specific treatment and rehabilitation to the developmentally disabled individuals, and not to a custodial placement.

Last, Dr. Bollinger wrote the customary disclaimers, distinguishing his forensic report from a purely clinical one.

The referenced individual was examined with reference to specific circumstances emanating from the incident in question, in accordance with the restrictive rules concerning an independent medical examination. It is, therefore, understood that no treatment was given or suggested, and that no doctor/patient relationship exists.

I aver that the information contained in this document was prepared by the undersigned and is the work of the undersigned. It is true to the best of my knowledge and information, and has not been modified by anyone other than the undersigned.

Please advise me if you have questions about this evaluation and report, or if you anticipate requiring additional services from me in connection with this matter.

Thank you very much.
Sincerely,
Curtis Bollinger, MD, MPH
Diplomate, American Board of Psychiatry and Neurology (P)
Certified, American Society of Addiction Medicine

Case Analysis and Outcome

In this case, Mr. Taylor's cognitive limitations and impairment were the basis for defense counsel's seeking professional mental health consultation/evaluation about Mr. Taylor's competency to have engaged in several different types of behavior relevant to his charges of child sexual abuse. The first of these—those of his criminal responsibility and alleged sexual abuse of his daughter—addressed the issue of past inferences about Mr. Taylor's mental state and psychiatric/neuropsychiatric/addiction medicine condition over a period of time during which he repeatedly engaged in the sexual activities. The issue in those situations is whether or not those inferences about Mr. Taylor's underlying mental state and psychiatric/neuropsychiatric/addiction medicine condition supported a criminal responsibility-reducing psychiatric defense, that is, legal insanity, diminished capacity, intoxication, or irresistible impulse, part of the applicable law in the jurisdiction.

The second time frame issue—Mr. Taylor's inferrable mental state and psychiatric/neuropsychiatric/addiction medicine condition surrounding Mr. Taylor's having waived his constitutional *(Miranda)* rights by giving a potentially inculpatory statement to police investigators—was cast differently. In that type of competency, the law required that for an individual to have competently waived constitutional rights, that waiver must be "knowing, voluntary, and intelligent."

The third time frame to be addressed in this evaluation is that of the present and reasonably foreseeable future, in terms of Mr. Taylor's competency to stand trial status. The consulting mental health professional's evaluation and opinion in this aspect of this matter, like that of the other two aspects of this evaluation, rely on inferences about Mr. Taylor's underlying mental state and psychiatric/neuropsychiatric/addiction medicine condition as of the time of the actual interview/examination, as well as on other sources of information upon which these types of evaluations are generally based (see Chapter 1).

After exploring all three of these areas and time frames, the consulting/evaluating mental health professional offered opinions supporting Mr. Taylor's having the cognitive capacity to be considered mentally competent by the court in all three areas, notwithstanding his clear and clinically significant cognitive impairment. In all three of these areas, to whatever extent Mr. Taylor's cognitive impairment and limited abilities may have affected his thought processes and behavior, they did not so adversely affect them (in this consultant/evaluator's opinion) as to support a formal court determination of incompetency in any of the three areas under consideration.

As a clinically informed and guided evaluation and report, the writer concluded with a recommendation for a clinical/therapeutic, and not strictly custodial, disposition for Mr. Taylor. From a humanitarian perspective, the court and prosecution agreed. However, the nature of Mr. Taylor's offenses and even the most liberal (but necessary, for the court) interpretation of applicable criminal law did not permit such a disposition. Mr. Taylor was ultimately sentenced to a lengthy term in state prison, by plea negotiation. The case did not go to trial, and in the final analysis, Dr. Bollinger's evaluation and report were of limited value and guidance to the court because of the strictness and rigidity of criminal law applicable to Mr. Taylor's offenses.

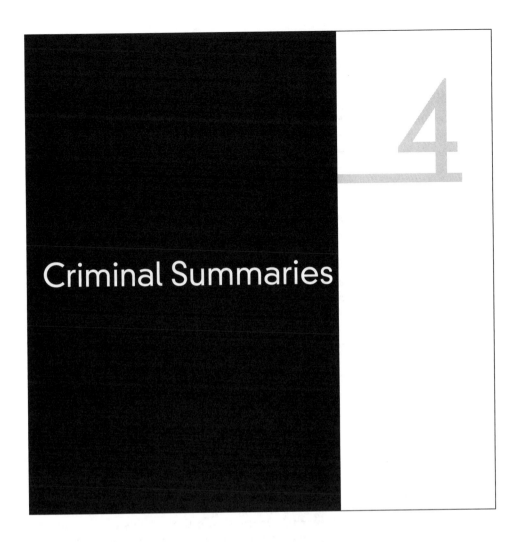

Criminal Summaries

The full range of possible criminal forensic mental health topics is vast, and covers all of the areas given in all of the time frames described in the applicable tables in Chapter 1. Although four full report examples of these types of cases are given in Chapter 3, time and space in this volume do not permit the presentation of examples of full reports of all of the potential types of criminal forensic mental health topics.

To make up for the necessarily limited range of criminal forensic mental health topics discussed as full reports in Chapter 3, this present chapter gives a series of additional excerpts from full reports. These excerpts are taken from the "Summary and Opinions" sections (that is, the final sections) of full reports from almost all of the topics presented in Table 1.2 of Chapter 1. Since this last section both summarizes the facts of the case and the forensic mental health expert's reasoning and opinions in the case, these brief accounts enable the reader to learn about a wider variety of criminal forensic mental health topics than is covered in the full detail of the four full reports from Chapter 3. In this way, we convey to the reader a broader range of forensic mental health topics in the criminal arena.

Violence: Not Guilty by Reason of Insanity (NGRI)/ Competent to Stand Trial (CST)

This defendant was arrested and indicted for the strangulation murder of a lover. Immediately after the killing the defendant fled the scene and was found barricaded in a hotel room several miles away. The individual's dysfunctional, marginal, and often nonproductive history included several criminal episodes and psychiatric hospitalizations where he was known to be noncompliant with reference to medications.

The overall evaluation of this individual included a determination, based on a review of all records available and several interviews, that the defendant was aware of the implications of the actions when the *Miranda* rights form was signed. Further, the inferences that could be drawn concerning the defendant's mental state and psychiatric/neuropsychiatric/addiction medicine condition at the time of the murder would support a court determination of any of the three potential criminal responsibility-reducing defenses, that is, legal insanity, diminished capacity, or intoxication. Additionally, in the opinion of the forensic psychiatrist, the defendant should be committed to a long term, but not to a custodial term, so that appropriate treatment could be provided. It was the belief of the psychiatrist that if adequate treatment and rehabilitation efforts were provided, the defendant would not be likely to act out again in a dangerous or violent way, even given the opportunity to do so.

Violence: NGRI

This individual was described as having a long-standing psychiatric history, most frequently diagnosed as schizophrenia, paranoid type, with periods of exacerbation and remission over the years. At the time of this evaluation, the individual was hospitalized in a mental institution several months after having beaten a parent to death in what was described as a drunken, psychotic rage.

In the view of the forensic psychiatrist, the individual showed good progress except for those times when level of privilege (LOP) status was reduced. It was felt by the psychiatrist that punishment for noncompliance through reduction in LOP status was not a positive or productive approach to treatment in this case. Additionally, the psychiatrist noted that the patient may be suffering from an underlying bipolar disorder, a possible cause of the irritability exhibited. It was recommended that appropriate medication, particularly a mood-stabilizing agent, be administered. Finally, since the individual did not appear to present a clinical picture of someone who was likely to act out in a dangerous or violent way, it was recommended that an LOP status be provided that would permit attendance at a local college as part of continuing therapy.

Violence: NGRI/CST

This defendant was indicted for the capital murder of an uncle and armed robbery of that victim's father. The defendant was evaluated using a wide variety of standardized and nonstandardized tests, interviews with relatives, review of all relevant and available records concerning the case, and interviews of the defendant. The defendant was described as having suicidal ideations, depression, and hallucinations, all of which resulted in psychiatric hospitalization while awaiting trial.

It was the opinion of the forensic psychiatrist, after conducting the evaluation (which included interviews with the defendant over a three-month period), that this individual was CST.

Violence: NGRI

This defendant-patient had a long-standing history of isolated living, psychotic-level psychiatric disorder, marginal adjustment to society in terms of relationships with others and work, and substance abuse (alcohol and marijuana, primarily) for what was likely self-medication of chronic dysphoria, delusional paranoid thoughts and ideation, and other such psychotic-level symptomatology. The defendant was characterized as a chronic psychotic-level psychiatric (schizophrenia, paranoid type). The criminal offense that resulted in arrest was drug use and possession.

While living an isolated existence, the defendant developed two related interests, first, a belief in the existence of UFOs and, second, in collecting weapons to defend against them. This collection included pipe bombs, gunpowder, and chemicals.

In the opinion of the forensic psychiatrist, the defendant was not aware that what was being done in terms of collecting the pipe bombs and associated paraphernalia was wrong and thus, the defense of NGRI would be available. Such a defense, however, was felt not to apply to the drug charge facing the defendant. As an alternative to incarceration, the psychiatrist recommended referral to a treatment setting with a long-term drug and alcohol rehabilitation program.

Violence: NGRI

The defendant was charged with the shotgun murder of a lover, and convicted of that and related offenses. The initial psychiatric evaluation opined that the defendant had experienced a dissociative event for the incident and, broadly speaking, was not acting in a purposeful and knowing manner at the time of the murder. A second forensic psychiatric opinion was requested.

It was the opinion of the second forensic psychiatrist who reviewed the relevant and available materials that based on the defendant's purposeful, goal-directed, complex, planned and executed, and sophisticated mental states and behaviors in connection with the shooting, along with the defendant's efforts to leave the scene, that the individual was sufficiently aware of what happened, even if there were two circumscribed periods of amnesia (dissociation) afterward, for the events themselves. The psychiatrist's opinion concluded with the statement that given the activities, behaviors, and mental states that, in terms of potentially applicable forensic psychiatric criminal defenses in this case, such as legal insanity, diminished capacity, and/or intoxication, none would apply.

Violence: NGRI/Diminished Capacity

The forensic psychiatrist in this case was asked for an opinion as to whether one or more of the jurisdiction's criminal responsibility-reducing defenses, such as legal insanity, diminished capacity, or intoxication, might be interposed. It was also requested that a determination be made as to whether the defendant was CST. The defendant-patient was charged with shooting a lover in the back four times with a handgun at a close range.

The forensic psychiatrist reviewed all relevant and available records and conducted a face-to-face meeting with the defendant. No opinion regarding the defendant's mental state as drawn in terms of inference was offered because of the lack of information provided by the defendant's mental state and psychiatric/neuropsychiatric/addiction medicine condition. At the time of the interview, the report held that the defendant was not CST.

Violence: NGRI

The patient-defendant in this case was indicted for the slaying of a spouse. At the time of this evaluation, the individual was incarcerated pending trial. There was a long history of prescribed medication use and, prior to the incident, ingestion of some alcohol. The defendant was known to be both irritable and angry with regard to the marital relationship.

In the opinion of the forensic psychiatrist, the individual, because of a state of intoxication with prescribed medications at the time of the slaying, combined with agitation and desperation with spouse and children, and the unlikely event that there was any intent to murder, was unable to form the specific intent to have engaged in a knowing and purposeful manner as otherwise required to commit the offense.

Violence: NGRI

This individual, at the time of the evaluation, was a patient in a psychiatric setting. The criminal offense was an arson in which a nephew of the defendant accidentally died. The individual was found NGRI. The patient has been institutionalized in hospitals and prisons for many years both before and after the arson. The patient held the belief that psychotropic medications being administered were the cause of psychiatric behavior.

The requested evaluation in this case centered on two points: first, to determine whether the defendant/patient had a current, substantial mental disorder that made the defendant/patient dangerous, and second, to ascertain whether the current medications being administered were correct, or if other medication should be forced; or if other treatments would be preferable, and, finally, if day passes and brief family visits would be beneficial.

In the opinion of the forensic psychiatrist, the patient clearly did suffer from a psychiatric disorder. Further, the patient was held to be on the correct treatment program and medications. A prevocational program was recommended; day passes, then overnight passes, and finally longer outpatient treatment were recommended as the individual showed benefit from increasingly less restrictive environments.

Violence: NGRI

This defendant had a virtually lifelong history of disruptive, psychiatric, and psychosocial problems, as well as a criminal history. The incident that led to this evaluation, and with regard to which the defendant was arrested, took place when, in an agitated and delusional state of mind, he mistakenly entered the home of another, believed that he was being poisoned, and requested help in a vague and confused way. A fight then ensued with the owner of the house, which resulted in the owner shooting the defendant and accidentally also shooting his own mother. The woman subsequently died as a result of the shooting.

It appeared that the defendant had a psychotic reaction to PCP (phencyclidine), which he had somehow ingested. This resulted in fear, feelings of being poisoned, delusional ideas about being Jesus Christ, and feelings of invulnerability, among other bizarre and unusual features manifested during the incident.

In the opinion of the forensic psychiatrist, the defendant, at the time of the incident, understood neither the nature and quality of the act perpetrated nor that it was wrong. The defendant was reported seeking help, not seeking to engage in criminal activity. It was also concluded that the defendant's mental state would support a determination of legal insanity and that the defendant was CST.

Violence: NGRI

The individual regarding whom this report was prepared had a long-standing history of psychotic-level psychiatric disorder and a concomitant history of psychiatric treatment including hospitalization and pharmacotherapy. The defendant's characteristic cycle involved stopping medications, becoming psychotically symptomatic, decompensating, requiring hospitalization and restabilization on medication, accomplishment of restabilization, and discharge to an outpatient facility, followed by noncompliance with medication. This individual, thus described, had an incident with the police arising from a routine traffic stop, which led to arrest and to this evaluation.

In the opinion of the forensic psychiatrist, this individual had become noncompliant with medication and thus bizarre behavior, the attempt to bury a dead animal found on the road with the subsequent traffic stop, was carried out in a mental state when the individual was not aware of the nature and quality of the act in which engaged and, that, by virtue of that lack of awareness, the individual did not know that the act was wrong.

The recommendation of the forensic psychiatrist was that a period of court-ordered supervision would be useful in providing clinical treatment and reducing the likelihood of another cycle of noncompliance/psychosis.

Sex Offender

The individual in this matter had been convicted of a sex offense some 30 years prior to this evaluation. The issue here involved a proposal by the state to have the individual placed in the Tier II level under that jurisdiction's *Megan's Law* provisions. A Tier II level would require community notification and placement of the individual's identity and offense history on the Internet. The individual protested this level and counsel arranged for a forensic psychiatric evaluation.

In the opinion of the expert, subsequent to a review of all relevant records and a meeting, the individual's stable history over a period of 15 years did not warrant Tier II level community notification. As noted in the report, the individual no longer possessed the energy, drive, urges, and desires to engage in sexually offensive behaviors and has not had such desires for many years.

Sex Offender

This defendant was diagnosed as suffering from bipolar disorder, manic, severe, with psychotic features, in addition to having a history of alcohol abuse. Following arrest, indictment, and incarceration for a sex offense involving two juveniles, this evaluation was conducted.

Based on available records, it was the opinion of the forensic psychiatrist that the offense in question that led to the arrest occurred during a time when the defendant was not on the proper medication. The result was that the defendant's judgment was poor, behavior was driven by uncontrolled symptomatology of the bipolar disorder, and thinking at the time was so distorted as to believe that the two juveniles were the criminal aggressors. In view of the defendant's mental condition, it was the opinion of the forensic psychiatrist that while the individual was aware of what was being done, there was no knowledge that it was wrong. The opinion was that the defendant had met the requirements of legal insanity, but was not functioning with diminished capacity at the time of the offense. Finally, in the opinion of the forensic psychiatrist, the defendant was CST.

Sex Offender

This defendant had a long history of bipolar disorder, psychiatric hospitalizations, and suicide attempts, that last of which caused a transfer to the most recent psychiatric hospitalization. The sexual offense involved the defendant's daughter. While incarcerated for that offense, the defendant attempted suicide by hanging.

Given the fact that the defendant admitted to the offense to the police and denied it to the forensic psychiatrist, it was impossible to determine the defendant's mental state at the time of the offense. If the defendant did not commit the offense charged, the mental state would not be relevant to the mental state and condition of someone who had committed such an offense. The report noted that the defendant was CST and the psychiatrist recommended that the defendant required constant ongoing psychiatric treatment regardless of the legal disposition of the case.

Sex Offender

This defendant, with a history of substance abuse, was arrested for prostitution. No evaluation was relevant with regard to legal insanity, diminished capacity, or intoxication given the nature of the case.

It was the opinion of the forensic psychiatrist that, as an alternative to a custodial setting, this defendant be placed in an inpatient/residential setting where psychiatric and chemical dependency needs would be addressed, and the prognosis for abstinence, sobriety, and recovery would be better addressed.

Violence: NGRI

The defendant in this case had been the victim of an abusive childhood. As an elementary school student, this individual was diagnosed as being dyslexic. Since childhood, the defendant had been placed, several times, in psychiatric hospitals, and was described as being a chronic psychotic-level patient, characteristically noncompliant with treatment and psychotropic medications.

The causative incident for this evaluation was that the defendant, reacting to what he perceived as the action of a friend in not providing comfort and security, placed a pipe bomb in the victim's automobile.

In the opinion of the forensic psychiatrist, the defendant did understand the nature of the act but did not understand that it was wrong. It was therefore the opinion that the defendant's inferrable mental state and psychiatric/neuropsychiatric condition would support a determination of legal insanity.

Violence: Intoxication

This individual, with a history of alcohol abuse, was arrested and indicted for manslaughter using a motor vehicle. This issue was whether the defendant could interpose the defense of intoxication.

The forensic psychiatrist, in order to determine the defendant's state of intoxication at the time of the offense, reviewed the relevant physiologic profile with reference to the ability on the part of this individual to absorb, distribute, metabolize, and excrete beverage alcohol. Additionally, it was necessary to determine the defendant's alcohol tolerance, largely through the actions and demeanor of the defendant immediately following the accident.

The resulting opinion was that the defendant was alcohol-tolerant and acted as though the BAC was lower than was the actual case. In setting out the opinion that the defense of intoxication would not be available, the psychiatrist opined that inferences about the defendant's underlying mental state and psychiatric/neuropsychiatric/addiction medicine (intoxication) condition during the period of time in question indicated that the defendant's ability to operate a motor vehicle safely was not clinically significantly impaired by the level of intoxication.

Domestic Violence

This individual, with a history of psychiatric hospitalization, was an NGRI patient showing progress toward discharge planning. An evaluation of status was deemed necessary following an incident involving the individual's elderly mother with whom there had been a long and tempestuous relationship.

In the opinion of the forensic psychiatrist who conducted the evaluation, the patient had shown clinical improvement and the incident in question should not negatively affect progress; therefore the recommendation was that the patient should be placed in the least restrictive environment possible to assist in a continued recovery and eventual reentry into the community. It was, however, also recommended that discharge planning should not be geared toward the patient living with the elderly mother, given their past history of incompatibility.

Domestic Violence

This individual was a resident of an assisted living facility and suffering from cognitive limitations and impairments. This court-appointed conservator requested the evaluation of this individual by a forensic psychiatrist. Several issues including the disposition of real property and the resolution of a criminal charge needed to be resolved in connection with this case. As a result, there was a determination needed regarding the individual's civil competency as well as one required in connection with CST.

The individual was described as having a long and troublesome marital relationship and a different, but still difficult, relationship with three sons. Based on a lengthy interview, it was the opinion of the forensic psychiatrist, with regard to the issue of civil competency, that the individual was not competent. Additionally, based on available medical records, the individual suffered from several conditions that included hypertension and dementia with behavioral disturbances. These factors, in the opinion of the forensic psychiatrist, contributed to the additional determination that the individual was not CST.

Malingering

The defendant in this case had a serious criminal record and at the time of this evaluation was in state prison on a charge of parole violation. The two questions in this case were, first, to determine if the defendant was CST and, second, to determine if the defendant's treatment at state prison was appropriate.

After conducting an interview, it was the opinion of the forensic psychiatrist that the defendant was CST. The psychiatrist stated in the case opinion that the defendant was malingering serious mental illness at the time of the interview/examination, such malingering being described in detail in the *Diagnostic and Statistical Manual of Mental Disorders-IV-Text Revision* (or *DSM-IV-TR*). Finally, it was recommended that then-ongoing treatment of the defendant be continued with some changes in medication considered. This recommendation was made on a guarded basis given the defendant's uncertain clinical condition and his inability to provide reliable information about the course of treatment.

Malingering

This defendant, indicted for murder, had a dysfunctional lifestyle and psychiatric problems, was a drug and alcohol abuser, and had a long adult criminal history. The central question in this case was whether the defendant was CST.

It was the opinion of the forensic psychiatrist that the defendant was CST and further that the defendant was a malingerer. The latter opinion was based on a comparison between two preview evaluations and a third, conducted five weeks later, where the defendant's mental condition had greatly (and incomprehensibly) deteriorated.

5

Full Civil Reports

In this chapter, we present a series of four full-length forensic civil psychiatric reports, modified and redacted to protect privacy, following the format described in Chapter 1. Like the criminal forensic reports in Chapter 3, these reports are a representative sample of the types of civil cases a forensic mental health expert would be likely to encounter in consulting to attorneys (plaintiff or defense) or the courts. They include:

- Personal Injury
- Sexual Harassment (Workplace)
- Professional Liability (Medical Malpractice)
- Civil Commitment (Mental Health Law)

After guiding the reader through the deconstructed reports with boldface commentary and discussion, we reproduce one of the four civil reports *(Holmes v. Moriarty Realty)* in full to give the reader a full picture of the final report.

Holmes v. Moriarty Realty

Case Overview: Personal Injury

The psychiatric expert sought by defense counsel was asked to evaluate the victim, Penelope Jane Holmes, in terms of the psychiatric/psychological responses and effects, if applicable, that the rape had on her as of the time of the psychiatric expert's examination (about 30 months after the rape), and the relationship of those responses and effects to the rape itself. In that respect, this evaluation is intended to focus on the *present* time frame (Table 1.1), and on the "damages" (a legal term) or "consequences; symptoms" (clinical terms) resulting from the traumatic event, more than on the time surrounding the rape itself. That characteristic distinction between criminal evaluation reports and civil evaluation reports, and others, will be developed further in the "Case Analysis and Outcome" sections of this chapter.

In keeping with the report format endorsed in this book (Table 1.4), the psychiatric expert in this matter (Dr. Selma J. Froyed, retained by defense counsel in this matter) began her report with identifying information about counsel's consultation referral and about the forensic mental health issues to be addressed in her evaluation. Dr. Froyed wrote the following report.

The Report

> This is the first (of four) reports of evaluations in civil law cases. This particular case presents a straightforward—if dramatic—example of a personal injury evaluation report that uses the full report format described in Chapter 1. In the introductory first section of the report, the writer lays out the nature and scope of the report, and the issues to be addressed in it. A clear and concise overview in that way is in keeping with the pointers given in Chapter 1: clear, concise, and jargon-free communication.

Following up on our telephone discussions and correspondence about the above-referenced matter, and based on the sources of information given below, I am writing you this report of my psychiatric/neuropsychiatric/evaluation of Ms. Penelope Jane Holmes in this matter.

This report is provided at your request, and is intended to give you my psychiatric/neuropsychiatric opinion—held with a degree of reasonable medical

> Dr. Froyed articulated the purpose, or goal, of this evaluation and report succinctly and simply. She also articulated the focus on present damages, and on a historical factor in Ms. Holmes's life involved in those damages.

probability—about Ms. Holmes's present mental state and psychiatric/neuro-psychiatric condition and its relationship, if applicable, to her experience of having been sexually assaulted (raped) on October 14, XXXX, in her apartment in Gotham City, Batstate, as described in further detail below.

At this early point in this present evaluation and report, I emphasize that the focus of this present evaluation and report is on Ms. Holmes's *present* psychiatric/neuropsychiatric condition, and is based on the sources of information described below. In this context, I note Ms. Holmes's history of an incident that occurred when she was 9 years old (to be discussed in further detail below), which resulted, among other points, in her feeling of distrust of mental health professionals, a distrust that she describes as having ramifications to the present in terms of her not having sought psychiatric/psychological help or counseling following the October 14, XXXX, incident in question. This and associated issues will be discussed in further detail below.

Next, the author gave an overview of the structure and scope of the report.

In this present report, after initially listing and discussing records and materials that I reviewed in connection with this evaluation and report, I will present and discuss Ms. Holmes's background and history as to the time of the October 14, XXXX, incident in question; and as to the time of my interview/examination of her in my office on December 20, XXXX, will present and discuss my psychiatric/neuropsychiatric observations and findings concerning Ms. Holmes from my interview/examination of her; will present and discuss my clinical diagnostic impressions of Ms. Holmes; and will conclude this report (in the section entitled "Summary and Opinions") with a discussion of Ms. Holmes's present psychiatric/neuropsychiatric condition and its relationship, again if applicable, to the October 14, XXXX, incident in question.

For further information and details about Ms. Holmes's background and history; her history up to the time of the October 14, XXXX, incident in question and its aftermath, to the present; and other such aspects of this matter, the reader is referred to applicable records and materials, described below.

The sources of information on which this present evaluation and report are based are as follows:

This case involved review of voluminous and extensive legal and medical records—called *discovery*, in legal parlance—for the forensic mental health evaluator. In cataloging, listing, and summarizing these records, part of the report becomes analogous to the trial attorney's trial notebook, as described in Chapter 1. This both enhances communication between the forensic evaluator and retaining counsel/court, and helps the evaluator to access records quickly and easily during testimony.

1. My review of copies of records and materials provided to me by your office in connection with this matter, as follows:

   a. A collection of employment/administrative records and materials pertaining to Ms. Holmes's present employment issues (she is employed with a fashion design firm in Gotham City, Batstate), psychiatric/neuropsychiatric or otherwise, pertaining to the October 14, XXXX, incident in question.

      For information and administrative/employment, payment, and related details contained in this collection, the reader is referred to it.

   b. "Interrogatories" (from defense to plaintiff) and "Answers to Interrogatories" (from plaintiff to defense) in this matter, dated July 10, XXXX, and undated, respectively. The interrogatories, for present purposes, are requesting a "Detailed description of injury or condition claimed to be permanent together with all present complaints" (Interrogatory 4), as well as a "Detailed description of nature, extent and duration of any and all injuries" (Interrogatory 3). The answer to Interrogatory 3 indicated that "I had bruises . . . I suffered emotional injuries. I continue to feel pain and discomfort . . . so I believe these injuries are permanent"; and the answer to Interrogatory 4 was as follows: "See prior answer. My present complaints include: I have a feeling of worthlessness . . . I feel dirty . . . I am very depressed and sad. I feel basically hopeless."

      Concerning the issue of treatment, Ms. Holmes's answer to Interrogatory 8 ("It's still being treated") addresses that issue: "I may see a therapist but right now I do not feel trust in anyone to do that."

      The answer to Interrogatory 2 gave a detailed account of the rape incident in Ms. Holmes's apartment in Gotham City during the early morning hours of October 14, XXXX. The reader is referred to that answer for further information and details.

   c. A collection of medical records and materials from Dr. Goodwin Bones (orthopedist), including clinical notes as well as a copy of chart entries and progress notes from Ms. Holmes's emergency department evaluation and treatment at the Gotham City Medical Center (GCMC; Gotham City, Batstate). Dr. Bones's notes for present purposes, to my reading, do not specifically discuss Ms. Holmes's sexual assault. However, "GCMC Emergency Department Nurses Notes" do.

      The "Multi-Disciplinary Assessment/Progress Notes" (Section 4) evaluation states the following:

      > Pt. [patient] tearful, but cooperative in answering questions appropriately. C/O [complains of] sexual assault and brought to ER by GCPD. +[present vaginal penetration] with penis. -anal penetration. -[no] oral contact/sex . . . Pt. stated she tried to wrestle with . . . assailant to "get away," but assailant had gun + and she "feared for her life."
      >
      > States assailant tied her wrists . . . Pt. states assailant lifted her shirt to expose her breasts, took off her underwear and shorts.

   d. A letter from Dr. Bones to Clarence Darrow, III, Esquire (Ms. Holmes's counsel in this matter), undated and forwarded to you by Mr. Darrow in a transmittal letter dated May 31, XXXX. Dr. Bones wrote about Ms. Holmes, saying she "came to my office on November 10, XXXX, for injuries as a result of an incident that had occurred on October 14, XXXX. Firstly, she was in a great deal of mental and emotional distress. I had to approach her with very gentle care because her body was in such a guarded and protective state. . . . She then had to seek other forms of treatment to address her needs. I feel that this incident has given her a real setback which she is slowly recovering from. . . . She came for a total of 14 visits."

e. A collection of criminal/legal/discovery records and materials from the Gotham City Police Department pertaining to the police response and investigation of the rape incident against Ms. Holmes of October 14, XXXX. Records and materials consisted of the Incident Reports from responding officers and other such records and materials.

To my reading, the summary of the incident in question, by Police Officer Theo Roosevelt, is the most detailed, as follows:

> Upon arrival the victim stated as she came out of her kitchen into her living room she observed a male with a dark hooded sweat shirt coming out of her bathroom. The actor and the victim began struggling; the actor then forced the victim into the bedroom, tied her hands behind her back, and covered her face with a shirt. When the victim was screaming the actor then retrieved the radio from the kitchen and placed it in the living room on the floor and played the music real loud.
>
> Actor then crawled up on top of the victim, pulled her shirt up kissing her breasts and pulled her panties and shorts down. The victim told the actor she was sick and he better have a condom. He stated, "Oh of course," and she believed he put it on. The actor then inserted his penis into her vagina. After completing the act the actor stated to the victim, "DON'T TELL ANYONE. I KNOW WHERE YOU LIVE. I'M GOING TO KILL YOU." Actor then left through the bedroom apartment window.

For further information contained in police reports and related records and materials contained in this collection, the reader is referred to it.

In all of these discussions and paraphrasing of records reviewed, criminal and clinical alike, Dr. Froyed summarizes those parts that are most relevant, in her view, for her evaluation and report, and for future testimony, should that be required.

---

f. A psychiatric evaluation report and C.V. for Marcus Welby, Jr., MD, in this matter, indicating that Ms. Holmes had been seen in consultation on July 1, XXXX. These two materials were sent under a transmittal letter to you from Mr. Darrow, dated August 10, XXXX.

In his report, Dr. Welby first noted that the purpose of the evaluation was "to evaluate her [Ms. Holmes's] psychiatric condition," and he next listed the five sets of records and materials that he had reviewed in connection with his evaluation. The "Description of Injury" section of the report, to my reading, was lengthy, and elaborated on summaries given, for example, in the police reports noted above. The reader is referred to those sections of Dr. Welby's report for details.

After discussing the events in the October 14, XXXX, incident in question of her subsequent evaluation at the GCMC, Dr. Welby wrote, "In the late morning, Ms. Holmes was able to leave the hospital. She and Vincent were escorted by a police detective to the SAVA Unit at the local precinct house in order for the incident to be recorded. She was again expected to describe the details of the rape, which was overwhelming. After approximately two hours, she could no longer deal with the stress. She became very angry at this point, so the police ended their query and drove Ms. Holmes and Vincent home. When she arrived at her apartment, Ms. Holmes found that most of the surfaces were covered with black fingerprint powder, and that the door to the apartment was taped . . . She went to visit with her childhood friend, who lives in northern Batstate, for a few weeks. Upon her return, she moved to another apartment. Though she would have preferred moving to another apartment complex, she and Vincent were not able to afford this type of a move."

Next in the report, Dr. Welby described Ms. Holmes's symptomatic responses to the incident in question from a psychiatric perspective, noting such symptomatology consistent with posttraumatic stress disorder (PTSD) as Ms. Holmes "continues to persistently reexperience the rape via recurrent and intrusive distressing recollections of the rape. She frequently experiences flashbacks of the rape, and continues to have illusions of 'shadows' of men in her apartment. . . . Numbing of general responsiveness is manifested via anhedonia, feelings of detachment and estrangement from others, a restricted range of affect, and a sense that life will encompass multiple strategies . . . a substantial decrease in appetites accompanied by gastrointestinal distress and weight loss, an extreme delay in sleep onset, which finally occurred when the sun began to rise, accompanied by sleeping into the early afternoon, nonrestorative sleep, psychomotor retardation, a sense of immobilization . . . excessive anxiety and worry about a number of issues that typically relate to trust, safety, vulnerability, and the future . . . panic attacks, which she continues to experience approximately twice a week. These attacks began when Ms. Holmes returned to work. The anticipatory anxiety regarding her ability to function effectively and cope with her sense of vulnerability may have been the precipitating factor for most of the attacks. Anticipatory anxiety for future attacks, and avoidant behavior secondary to the attacks, has not developed."

On Mental Status Examination, Dr. Welby noted that "it took time for Ms. Holmes to begin speaking about the rape, due to the intensity of her distress regarding its recollection. Mood was clearly despondent. Affect was consistent with mood, with intermittent tearfulness noted. When discussing the details of the rape, Ms. Holmes appeared to be experiencing flashbacks, which she acknowledged were occurring. Cognition appeared intact."

Next, in his report, Dr. Welby described Ms. Holmes's account of her own personal and developmental history (also discussed below). For present purposes, comparing Ms. Holmes's description of herself before and after the incident in question, Dr. Welby wrote that "Ms. Holmes described herself, prior to the rape, as a physically and socially active woman, who enjoyed her work, her home, and her relationships. She enjoyed movies, dancing, walking through the streets of Gotham City, being with friends, writing poetry, and attending a writer's group. Her desire to help others led her to volunteer with a group for foreign students. . . . Ms. Holmes has no personal history of prior psychiatric illness or intervention, nor a family history for psychiatric illness. She did not serve in the military. She has not been involved in prior litigations. . . . After the rape, she went into a 'black hole,' 'withdrawing into a cell' and feeling unable to bring herself back to life. She describes that every day was tremendously painful, and that her sense of self was broken. Feeling terrified of being alone, she pleaded with Vincent to resign from work and stay home with her to protect her, which he did not do. Vincent continued to work. She began to irrationally blame him for not being at home when the intruder broke in and, therefore, not being able to prevent the rape. She then developed a fear that Vincent would not be available when she needed him the most, which precipitated unrealistic rage, causing her to end their relationship multiple times . . . .

"Prior to the rape, Ms. Holmes described that she and Vincent had wonderful sexual intimacies. She was proud of her body and comfortable with her sexuality. She felt free, and very much enjoyed lovemaking with Vincent. After she was raped, it took one year before Ms. Holmes was willing to be sexually intimate. Her present sexual intimacies now occur approximately once per month, and no longer feel the same. She states, 'I'm no longer the same person.'"

Subsequently, "Ms. Holmes was informed that the rapist was apprehended. The semen left on her sheet provided the deoxyribonucleic acid (DNA) evidence to track him down. Ms. Holmes felt empowered by having realized at the time of the rape that this would be the clue to his identity and apprehension. She also felt a sense of justice. Though she initially felt a sense of relief that he could no longer kill her, this did not have any impact on her extreme sense of fear and vulnerability."

In terms of employment, Dr. Welby wrote, "Ms. Holmes realized that it was unhealthy for her to be isolated and dysfunctional, although she felt too vulnerable and inadequate after the rape to resume her employment. Ms. Holmes finds she's very forgetful, that her mind will go blank and that she no longer can register information as she did before. Though previously she had been dynamic in problem solving, she now feels overwhelmed. Her sense of inadequacy is pervasive, as is her sadness. Ms. Holmes relates that luckily, her co-workers and supervisors have been very supportive of her. A co-worker gave her a car, but she was too frightened to drive, due to her insecurities, and feared that she would get into a fatal accident. Instead, she commutes by public transportation . . . which is a long trip."

In terms of diagnostic considerations, Dr. Welby gave the following using the nosology and format of the *DSM-IV-TR* (also described below):

Axis I (Posttraumatic Stress Disorder):

Major depressive disorder, single episode severe, without psychotic features.

Axis II

No diagnosis.

Axis III

No general medical condition.

Axis IV (Psychosocial and Environmental Stressors):

Unsafe home environment in which rape occurred, causing severe depression, immobilization, and interpersonal conflict.

Axis V (Global Assessment Functioning [GAF]):

Score of 52.

Finally, in terms of "Treatment Recommendations," Dr. Welby recommended "a combination of pharmacotherapy and psychotherapy for Ms. Holmes's treatment." She also noted that, "Unfortunately, due to this sense of vulnerability and feared victimization, Ms. Holmes has not felt able to commit to psychiatric treatment for fear if she were to open herself to a therapeutic process, it would leave her vulnerable to the physician." (As discussed in further detail below, when Ms. Holmes related her history to me she indicated her sense of concern about a repeat betrayal by a treating psychiatrist, as she had previously experienced when she was 9 years old, and as also discussed above.)

Dr. Welby's "Impression" in this report, was that "aforementioned psychiatric illnesses are directly related to and caused by the rape that occurred on October 14, XXXX. Due to the intensity of the trauma, and the severity of the subsequent psychiatric deterioration, permanent psychiatric sequelae are to be expected."

Dr. Froyed discussed Ms. Holmes's deposition in this matter as she did other records and materials. She excerpted those parts most relevant to her evaluation and report, paraphrasing and discussing them.

g. A copy of the transcript of Ms. Holmes's deposition in this matter, taken on July 14, XXXX.

To my reading, the content of this deposition reiterates and enlarges on a number of points made in other records and materials (such as police reports, GCMC emergency department evaluation notes for Ms. Holmes, and other such documentation).

For present purposes, in terms of her psychiatric/neuropsychiatric condition and its relationship to the rape incident, and subsequent treatment, Ms. Holmes indicated that she had contacted a crisis hotline following the rape and had spoken with individuals on that hotline twice, and that she had seen Dr. Welby for an evaluation, but was not involved in any psychiatric treatment following the incident in question. She also indicated that when she was 9 years old, she had "an experience in school a long time ago" that influenced her decision not to seek psychiatric treatment following the rape incident in question.

Ms. Holmes testified in her deposition that she "was like 9 years old and we had a psychologist at school and I shared some very private things with her and she went and told the principal and I was expelled from school. . . . I was living with my great aunt and two neighbors came on to me and were trying to seduce me every night late at night after everybody went to sleep, and although there was never a sexual interaction, there was a very sexual nature to it and I was—I felt totally trapped and I went to look for help to the psychologist of the school. The psychologist told the principal about what I shared with her, which I thought was confidential, and out of that, I was expelled from school, I was humiliated, my mother was humiliated, my family was—I was stuck for at least more than seven months at home totally ashamed and trapped out of trying to reach for help and being, like, open and vulnerable with authority about the issue and totally being betrayed and that's why I haven't been able to reach psychological help because even though I know I need it and even though I must do it, I can't bring myself to do it, so that's why I keep postponing and I keep putting it off to call professional help regarding this issue."

In terms of the consequences of the October 14, XXXX, rape incident in question, Ms. Holmes also testified in her deposition that "I totally lost my senses of self, my self-confidence, my self-esteem, I feel broken and fragmented, I feel unsafe in general, I don't have certainty about the things that I used to be certain about, like my career and my emotional life. My boyfriend . . . is impacted by this incident. . . . Because there is a part of me that blames him for not being there when this happened, as much as I've tried to let go of that and be rational about it that he has nothing to do with it, I keep coming back to that and feeling unprotected with him and it leaves me very uncertain about my future with him. . . . I feel paranoid and I was very—before the incident, I was very free to be outside with people and now I feel that I'm always looking who's around me and feeling like anybody could harm me, which it was not like before that. . . . In my job now, I am noticing that my memory is really bad now. I'm not as sharp as I used to be, and just little, basic simple tasks, and that accompanied by a feeling of inadequacy, not being capable and just feeling ugly. . . . Embarrassed, I feel embarrassed and guilty and ashamed also. . . . I had questions about my career, I was—but no, than that no . . . whether I chose the right thing, whether I would be doing that for the rest of my life or not, those kinds of questions . . . ."

Ms. Holmes also commented in her deposition that in terms of her current status, "Things have gotten better. I'm spending more time with friends, I'm forcing myself to be with people and reach family members that I haven't in a long time so that's been helping me . . . crying? . . . know I am eating better . . . I had diarrhea for a month after the incident and everything that I ate, I vomited, I felt so sick . . . at least 20 pounds . . . [weight loss] . . . Yeah [her weight returned] . . . ."

In terms of additional consequences of the incident in question, Ms. Holmes, ended: "Sexually. I am not the same person sexually as I was before . . . not as frequent and also, I'm very suppressed now, where I was not before . . . we've [she and Vincent] been broken up since December on and off a couple of times and finally it happened like three weeks ago. . . . I don't go out as much. I used to go dancing late at night, I used to—once I went camping by myself. I could not dare to do that now. I am always afraid now and I wasn't before. . . . Socially, I was never awkward and I was very social before and now I'm very self-conscious when I'm with people, like, I—I feel that I had this big secret that I am imprisoned by and I feel that I am less than everybody else."

For further information and details contained in this deposition transcript, the reader is referred to it.

Dr. Froyed next listed and briefly discussed the additional (i.e., not documents or written records and materials) sources of information on which her evaluation and report of Ms. Holmes were based.

---

2. My psychiatric/neuropsychiatric/addiction medicine interview/examination of Ms. Penelope Holmes in my office on November 30, XXXX, which interview/examination included the administration and subsequent scoring and interpretation of a series of standardized and nonstandardized psychological, chemical dependency, and related tests and inventories, as described below;

3. As part of my psychiatric/neuropsychiatric interview/examination of Ms. Holmes, the administration and subsequent scoring and interpretation of a series of standardized and nonstandardized psychological, chemical dependency, and related tests and inventories, as follows:

   a. The Minnesota Multiphasic Personality Inventory, 2nd Edition, or MMPI-2;
   b. The Millon Clinical Multiaxial Inventory, 3rd edition, or MCMI-III;
   c. The Beck Depression Inventory, 2nd edition, or BDI-II;
   d. The Addiction Assessment (nonstandardized) Questionnaire;
   e. The Michigan Alcohol Screening Test, or MAST;
   f. The Drug Abuse Screening Test, or DAST;

g. The Alcohol Use Disorders Identification Test, or AUDIT;

h. The Mini-Mental State Examination, or MMSE;

i. The Cognitive Capacity Screening Examination, or CCSE; and

j. The Past Medical History (nonstandardized) Questionnaire; and

4. My knowledge, background, training, and experience in psychiatry and neuropsychiatry, addiction medicine, and forensic psychiatry, and—for present purposes—my work and experience in occupational psychiatry.

The "History" section of this full report draws a distinction between Ms. Holmes's unremarkable and stable preincident background and her prominent psychiatric symptomatology following the incident. This illustrates the role of the forensic evaluator in addressing damages (in legal parlance: Clinicians might use the terms *consequences* or *symptomatology* resulting from the injury or incident in the same way), but not *liability* (the legal question of whether or not the defendant in a civil case acted illegally or otherwise inappropriately in allegedly somehow harming, or damaging, the plaintiff) in the forensic evaluation. In this particular case, careful and frequent telephone communication—an important pointer in the expert/attorney or court/attorney relationship—helped to clarify this distinction for both.

History

Ms. Penelope (Penny) Jane Holmes, is a 26-year-old (DOB: January 26, XXXX) single (never married; Ms. Holmes has a boyfriend, Vincent, West, CPA, age 32, whom she has been dating since August) white female, currently living in a rented private home in Gotham City, where the rape in question occurred on October 14, XXXX.

Ms. Holmes described a psychologically traumatic event when she was 9 years old (see above), which she said resulted in her distrust of psychologists and therapists for a period of time, but not in permanent psychological consequences of sequelae.

Ms. Holmes has been employed with a fashion design firm in Gotham City, a position that she had held for several years after her graduation from the University of Greenstate, where she majored in art and art history. Ms. Holmes had been born and raised in rural and suburban Greenstate, and had never ventured outside that state for longer than one week until she relocated to Gotham City "to try something new" (her words). In addition to her work with the design firm, Ms. Holmes also was employed part-time at an upscale restaurant "to make ends meet" (her words).

In terms of her own personal and psychosocial background and history, Ms. Holmes is an only child, born and raised in Greenstate in what she described as a "very happy" childhood. Both of Ms. Holmes's parents, Sherwood Holmes and Jane Holmes, died at the ages of 55 and 53, respectively, in XXXX, when Ms. Holmes was in her senior year at college. To the best of her knowledge, both of

Ms. Holmes's parents were healthy, and she herself was not aware of any family history of serious medical, psychiatric, or related such problems, even in her elderly grandparents and extended family.

Ms. Holmes described her childhood, adolescence, and young adult years as "very happy" ones, in which she enjoyed college, did well academically, was popular, and enjoyed a number of social and extracurricular activities. While in college and for a period of time before meeting Vincent West, her present boyfriend, Ms. Holmes had several intimate heterosexual relationships. She then met Vincent at a business lunch, and they started dating immediately and exclusively, but not living together (in that regard, Ms. Holmes described that her "independence is very important to me").

At this point in the report, Dr. Froyed discusses Ms. Holmes's account of the incident in question, quoting that account and emphasizing that it may be one of several to which it may be compared.

With the above background and history, Ms. Holmes's account to me (during my interview/examination of her)—an account that may be compared with others, described above and elsewhere in records and materials available for review—about the rape incident of October 14, XXXX, was as follows:

Vincent was working late, we went to a movie, and I took the subway home, by 1:00 A.M. I opened the door, it was hot. I opened the windows, wide open, to the bathroom, and kitchen. I changed clothes to light clothes, and started to wash dishes. I got wrapped up, did cleaning. I had a bag of garbage. I looked at the clock, 3:00 A.M. I was in the kitchen the entire time. I grabbed garbage and saw a shadow go from the bedroom to the bathroom. I thought it was Vincent. It had to be.

I started toward the door. A man jumped me from the back, and I started screaming. He covered my head with something. I was on the floor struggling, wrestling. "This is not going to happen to me." I couldn't turn over. He tried to asphyxiate me, strangle me, then I stopped. Then I said, "Why are you killing me?" He stopped, and I tried to wrestle. No go. His body is on top of me, torso and head. He took out a gun, I thought my life was in danger. I said, "Don't hurt me." He said, "If you do anything, I'll kill you."

Tied my hands behind my back, stood me up, walked me into the bedroom, sat me on my bed against the wall. I asked him, begged, just go. I tried to convince him there was nothing there. He said, "Where is the money?" It was a stupid apartment to break into. How old are you? "Early twenties." "You don't have to do this." He went into the kitchen when he put me onto the bed, got a boom-box from the kitchen to drown out my screams. Then he comes close, said, "I came here to take something." He kissed my neck. I knew he'd rape me. I screamed. He undressed me, my skirt, kissed my breasts, forced me, I begged him, fought, he raped me. I don't remember if I fought right then. I remembered he's untied me, waited five minutes. He threw my cell phone on the bed. I called 911 on the cell, was told not to clean or shower. Went to the window, he was gone, he'd untied me then. I didn't want to tell Vincent, not to trouble us.

The police came, questioned me in the kitchen. To the hospital, in an ambulance, I was a mess, crying, confused. I told the female ambulance attendant not to tell Vincent, she said I shouldn't go through this alone. She called him, he arrived a few hours later. A crisis protocol for him, too. A female detective drove me to the apartment, I showered, then slept through the afternoon. Vincent stayed there for two nights. There was a trace of DNA on the sheets, they eventually found the perpetrator. I was happy, no stalking, he said he'd kill me if I told anybody.

At this point in the report, Dr. Froyed continues Ms. Holmes's history following the rape incident.

After that, by her account, Ms. Holmes remained out of work for an extended period of time, indicating that, "I couldn't go back to my job, felt inadequate, couldn't leave the apartment much, felt horrible. I forced myself monthly to send a resume on the Internet. I stayed in the apartment two or three months."

Several months after the rape incident in question, Ms. Holmes was able to return to both of her previous jobs ("My bosses were very understanding and sympathetic. They were both women"). She described her necessary ADLs [Activities of Daily Living] as getting up early in the morning, showering and dressing and preparing her morning coffee, commuting to her principal job by subway, putting in a full day of work from about 8:00 A.M. to about 5:00 A.M., and feeling "better since I began to work again, less of a sense of inadequacy . . . simple tasks take a long time, I sometimes feel paranoid about work . . . get home in about two hours, with Vincent, shower, cook, check my e-mail, go to bed after the 11:00 P.M. news. Noises bother me, sex with Vincent still bothers me."

Next, Dr. Froyed addresses Ms. Holmes's account of the damages, in legal parlance, or clinical symptomatology resulting from the rape incident.

In terms of psychiatric symptomatology that Ms. Holmes attributes to the rape incident in question, she told me during my interview/examination of her that "concentration is down, like I'm another person. I cry easily, there's sadness and disbelief. I pull out my hair, have moments of madness, sex is still a problem with Vincent, used to be every day. We talk about moving in together and getting married and getting a place together. I haven't missed work, but I daydream at work in the design business, not waitressing."

Ms. Holmes's reasons for initiating the civil lawsuit in this matter, in the context of its relationship to her present psychiatric condition, she told me that she had made that decision "immediately, within the week. Before the incident, I knew there were break-ins, problems with security and heat. It's not right. I don't want that to happen to anybody else. I saw ads for attorneys, and I called them."

Concerning Ms. Holmes's "Three Wishes" (an informal psychological projective technique), she told me that they were to "erase my memory and be as innocent as I once was, feel happy, satisfied, fulfilled ... make up my mind about Vincent."

Finally, Ms. Holmes's rating of herself (on a scale of 0 to 10, in which 0 represents the worst she has ever felt, and the worst she has ever functioned, and 10 represents the best she has ever felt and the best she has ever functioned), Ms. Holmes gave various estimates for various important periods of her life. For example, she rated herself at 8 on the scale during her childhood and adolescence (not identifying very high or very low points during those years); 9 during her years as a student at the University of Vermont; 9 at obtaining her work in fashion design; 4 as she realized that she needed an extra job to "make ends meet" (see above); 8 at meeting and dating Vincent; 0 at the time of the rape incident in question; 6 currently in terms of her relationship with Vincent; and 5 as of the time of my interview/examination of her, in an overall sense. Ms. Holmes commented in response to my specific question that she would expect to be "maybe a 7 or 8 out of 10" when the above-referenced matter is resolved and she no longer has to contend with the exercises and activities associated with the case, as reminders to her of the rape incident in question.

As with any clinical or clinically based psychiatric/psychological report, the next two sections of this report present observations, findings, and clinical impressions from the interview/examination. This clinical focus on the present emphasizes Ms. Holmes's clinical status and condition as of the time of the actual interview/examination, and underscores the damages aspect of the forensic evaluation. It also lays the groundwork for the "Summary and Opinions" section of the report.

Mental Status (Psychiatric) Examination

This revealed a well-developed, well-nourished white female who was casually dressed in a green dress, a light coat, and women's boots, and who was neatly groomed with blonde hair.

I introduced myself to her, ascertained her understanding of the purpose and scope of the interview/examination, and advised her of the likelihood non-confidential nature of the evaluation. She told me this was acceptable to her. We then proceeded with the interview/examination.

Throughout the interview/examination, Ms. Holmes was pleasant and cooperative, and initially shy and reticent. As time went on, however, she appeared to become more comfortable and less inhibited to the interview/examination situation, her range affect increased, and she became more interactive with me. Throughout the interview/examination, in my view, Ms. Holmes was forthcoming, pleasant, and cooperative. Throughout this interview/examination, there was no indication of severe affective disorder or symptomatology (such as severe depression, mania, or suicidality), although Ms. Holmes did speak about a number of sad themes in her life, especially after the October 14, XXXX, rape incident in question. Similarly, there was no indication of thought disorder or psychotic processes or symptomatology (such as hallucinations, delusions, loosening of associations, and so forth) during this interview/examination.

> Since forensic mental health evaluation may not be confidential or privileged between the evaluator and the evaluee, it is important to point that out to evaluees at the beginning of the interview/examination, and to obtain their permission and consent to proceed. Some mental health professionals (like this writer) obtain such written consent with a formal instrument, analogous to obtaining informed consent to medical or surgical procedures; others do not. In criminal defense cases, it is ultimately defense counsel who decides whether the defense expert's opinion and report will be used, as an extension of a defendant's "right to remain silent." In prosecution-retained and court-appointed forensic mental health evaluations, in contrast, the defendant, in effect, has waived his or her privilege in previously offering a psychiatric defense, which may be explored by a prosecution and/or court-appointed expert. Therefore, no privilege or confidentiality applies to the evaluation and report, which are then made available to the defense, the prosecution, and the court.

Cognitively, Ms. Holmes was alert and oriented in all parameters (time, person, place, and circumstances of and reasons for this interview/examination, including her awareness that there would be no privacy or confidentiality between us associated with this interview/examination; this last point was acceptable to her), and her completion of the two standardized cognitive screening tests (the MMSE and the CCSE). Both test results were unremarkable and not indicative of severe organicity or cognitive impairment. Ms. Holmes's general discussion was consistent, in my view, with her level of life experience and formal education as a liberal arts college graduate.

> The use of standardized and nonstandardized testing and inventories is discussed in Appendix C. Dr. Froyed used tests to expand her knowledge and information about Ms. Holmes in general, and to survey her about areas already discussed (such as chemical dependency) using another (pencil-and-paper questionnaire) format.

Ms. Holmes's responses to the several standardized and nonstandardized psychological, chemical dependency, and related tests and inventories—beginning with the MMPI-2—yielded results that were considered invalid because: "There are indications that the test-taker answered randomly to many of the items without regard to their content. The profile appears invalid since it has not been completed properly. Little to no weight should be granted to the following interpretive information" (as described in the "Test-Taking Behavior" section of the computer-generated "Comprehensive Report" for this test).

On the other hand, the computer-generated "Interpretive Report" for Ms. Holmes's completion of the Millon Clinical Multiaxial Inventory, 3rd edition (MCMI-III), was described in that report as valid, in which "On the basis of the test data, it may be assumed that the patient is experiencing a severe mental disorder." That said, possible diagnoses for this set of results included "Major Depression (recurrent, severe, without psychotic features)," "Posttraumatic Stress Disorder," and "Adjustment Disorder With Mixed Anxiety and Depressed Mood" (as described in the "Possible Diagnoses" section of this report).

Consistent with Ms. Holmes's reported and described history of lack of problems in the area of alcohol and substance abuse, her responses to the several chemical dependency tests and inventories (the Addiction Assessment Questionnaire, the Michigan Alcohol Screening Test [MAST], the Drug Abuse Screening Test [DAST], and the Alcohol Use Disorders Identification Test [AUDIT]) were all indicative of no problems, past or present, in these areas.

Finally, Ms. Holmes's completion of the "Past Medical History" questionnaire indicated an individual in generally good health, not presently (or in the past) taking psychotropic medications or involved in psychiatric treatment, and without a prior history of psychiatric or other major medical problems.

In Ms. Holmes's completion of the "Diagnostic Criteria for PTSD" as presented in the *DSM-IV-TR*, she did not endorse either of the two "A" Diagnostic Criteria, although she did endorse them in her discussion of the October 14, XXXX, rape incident in question, during my interview/examination of her. These two criteria require that, "The person has been exposed to a traumatic event in which both of the following were present: (1) The person experienced, witnessed, or was confronted with an event or events that involved actual or threatened death or serious injury, or a threat to the physical integrity of self or others . . . (2) The person's responses involved intense fear, helplessness, or horror." In terms of Ms. Holmes's responses to other symptomatology in these diagnostic criteria, she endorsed fewer currently than had been the case within six months of the incident itself.

Anticipating the "Summary and Opinions" section of the report, this next section pulls together all of the preceding sections, giving a succinct description of Ms. Holmes's multiaxial diagnoses, with the nosology and format of the widely used and generally accepted *DSM-IV-TR*, as discussed earlier.

Clinical Diagnostic Impressions

In keeping with the current diagnostic nomenclature and format of the *Diagnostic and Statistical Manual of Mental Disorders, Fourth Edition, Text Revision* (2000), of the American Psychiatric Association, clinical diagnostic impressions for Ms. Holmes can be presented as follows:

Axis I (Clinical Disorders):

1. Major depression, single episode, recurrent, without psychotic features.
2. Posttraumatic stress disorder, chronic.

Axis II (Personality Disorders):

No diagnosis.

Axis III ("General Medical Conditions"):

Ms. Holmes appears to be in generally good medical condition, without indications of active, acute, chronic, or ongoing medical problems or conditions requiring medical attention or treatment.
In this context, however, I note Ms. Holmes's stating a need for psychiatric
treatment for problems and symptomatology associated with the October 14, XXXX, rape incident in question, despite her unwillingness to
be involved in such treatment.

Axis IV (Psychosocial and Environmental Problems):

As a practical clinical matter, Ms. Holmes's main present "Psychosocial and
Environmental Problems" relate to symptomatology associated with
the October 14, XXXX, rape incident in question, and its aftermath.
Otherwise, by her account, she has a supportive relationship with a
boyfriend, is gainfully employed and hardworking, has adequate housing, has resumed sexual activities with her boyfriend (although, by her
account, not to the pre-rape incident level), and has a sufficient educational background to employ her in professional work that she finds
enjoyable and fulfilling, if not sufficiently financially rewarding.
These and "Problems related to interactions with the legal system,"
specifically referring to exercises and activities associated with
the above-referenced lawsuit and its periodic reminders and associations to her of the October 14, XXXX, rape incident in question,
constitute, in my view, Ms. Holmes's main "Environmental and Psychosocial Problems" at this point. In that regard, Ms. Holmes herself estimated that her "self-rating" (see above) will be higher for her
once the above-referenced lawsuit has been resolved.

Axis V (Global Assessment of Functioning [GAF]):

A GAF Scale score of 60–70 signifying mild-to-moderate impairment and
symptomatology, in my opinion, applies here.

Summary and Opinions

Ms. Penelope Jane Holmes is a 26-year-old (DOB: January 26, XXXX) white female, educated and trained in areas of fashion and design, currently employed
in that capacity with a firm in Gotham City, Batstate, and currently involved
with her boyfriend, "Vincent," with whom she has had what she described as an
on-and-off relationship since they first started dating in May of XXXX.

As with the four criminal reports, this last section of this civil report—"Summary and Opinions"—summarizes a great deal of data in a concise and persuasive way. The predominantly neutral and objective language of the preceding sections is modified in this section, since it is here that the forensic evaluator expresses a forensic opinion—"based on a degree of reasonable medical—or psychological, or scientific—probability or certainty"—about the forensic issue or issues to be addressed in the evaluation. The opinion should be presented convincingly and persuasively: The forensic mental health evaluator is an advocate for his/her opinion, and not for any party.

With that background, Ms. Holmes was involved in the rape episode at her apartment in Gotham City during the early morning hours of October 14, XXXX, as described above and elsewhere in records and materials available for review in this matter. Following that incident, Ms. Holmes was evaluated on an emergency basis at the GCMC, and on occasions after that, made calls to a local hotline for counseling and support. She has not been involved in psychiatric treatment since that time, notwithstanding her acknowledgment that such treatment would be clinically indicated for her. She also remained out of work for an extended period of time after the incident in question, eventually returning to her present job.

Ms. Holmes's not having been involved in psychiatric or psychological treatment following the rape incident is an important aspect of Dr. Froyed's later characterization of her as a "survivor."

With this background and history, Ms. Holmes instituted the above-referenced lawsuit against her apartment owners. In the context of that lawsuit, your office arranged for this present second opinion (my characterization, a second opinion to that of Dr. Marcus Welby, described above) to explore the issue of Ms. Holmes's present psychiatric/neuropsychiatric condition and its relationship, if so, to her rape experience of October 14, XXXX.

The sources of information on which this present evaluation and report are based; Ms. Holmes's background and history leading up to the time of the rape incident in question; and then to the time of my interview/examination of her in this matter; my psychiatric/neuropsychiatric observations and findings concerning Ms. Holmes; and my clinical diagnostic impressions of Ms. Holmes are all as described above and elsewhere in records and materials available for review in this matter. That information will not be repeated in this section of this report.

Ms. Holmes's present psychiatric/neuropsychiatric condition, with associated diagnoses and levels of functioning, are as described above. While I do not significantly disagree, to my reading, with Dr. Welby's formulation of Ms. Holmes's present situation, I note that in the context of her life in general,

> At this point in the "Summary and Opinions" section, Dr. Froyed departs from the largely historical nature of her writing, and begins to present and elaborate on her opinions about reported damages to Ms. Holmes resulting from the rape.

Ms. Holmes's present self-rating (see above) is not very much different from self-ratings at other various points in her life (some of which have been psychologically traumatic for her); and that her own estimate of this rating as well as her endorsement of fewer symptoms in the Diagnostic Criteria of PTSD (since the time of the incident itself) shows improvement and amelioration in her clinical condition since the time of the incident itself. In that sense, as a "survivor" (my word; see above), Ms. Holmes may be considered to have "survived" the immediate and longer-term trauma of the October 14, XXXX, rape incident at issue.

In that vein, I note Dr. Welby's recommendation for psychotherapy and pharmacotherapy for Ms. Holmes. Ms. Holmes herself agreed that such treatment would be desirable for her. However, despite the advisability of such treatment for her, Ms. Holmes has managed to do as well as she has been doing—personally, professionally, socially, and with her boyfriend—without such help. This underscores her being a survivor, in my view. As contemplated by Dr. Welby, effective psychiatric treatment would likely help with Ms. Holmes's self-esteem, work-related symptomatology (e.g., her perception of memory problems), and her overall well-being: I agree that Ms. Holmes would be well advised to become involved in such treatment, but also note her current good functioning without such treatment.

> In this final substantive paragraph, Dr. Froyed succinctly presents her expert opinion in this matter, emphasizing her characterization of Ms. Holmes as a survivor.

Putting these various points together, it is my psychiatric/neuropsychiatric opinion—held with a degree of reasonable medical probability—that while Ms. Penelope Jane Holmes has experienced PTSD and other psychiatric problems as a result of the rape incident of October 14, XXXX, her response to that incident has been influenced and informed by her prior experience (referring, for example, to Ms. Holmes's self-ratings at various points in her life, both before and after the October 14, XXXX, incident in question); that notwithstanding that incident and its aftermath, Ms. Holmes has been able to continue her relationship with her boyfriend, Vincent, and to obtain work and thereby become independent in her day-to-day functioning again; that Ms. Holmes has been able to achieve these gains without psychiatric treatment and/or psychopharmacotherapy; and that, in sum, Ms. Holmes's status as a survivor (see above) has permitted her to do as well as she has been able to do, despite the rape incident itself and her lack of specific treatment or therapy after the incident to address the consequences and sequelae of that incident.

Finally, in the context of this present evaluation and report, I reiterate Ms. Holmes's perception that the stresses and reminders of exercises and activities associated with the litigation in this matter, which remind her and reinforce her feelings about the incident itself, once concluded, will permit her to move on and to increase her perception (i.e., her self-rating) in terms of her overall level of functioning and happiness.

> **Last, Dr. Froyed wrote the customary disclaimers, distinguishing her forensic report from a purely clinical one.**

The referenced individual was examined with reference to specific issues emanating from the original situation, in accordance with the restrictive rules concerning an independent medical examination. It is, therefore, understood that no treatment was given or suggested and that no doctor/patient relationship exists.

I aver that the information contained in this document was prepared by the undersigned and is the work of the undersigned. It is true to the best of my knowledge and information and has not been modified by anyone other than the undersigned.

Please advise me if you have questions about this present evaluation and report, or if you anticipate requiring additional services from me in connection with this matter.

Thank you very much.

Selma J. Froyed, MD

Case Analysis and Outcome

Referring to Table 1.1, this evaluation focuses on Dr. Froyed's inferences about the present psychiatric/neuropsychiatric/addiction medicine effects on Ms. Holmes resulting from the October 14, XXXX, rape incident in question. In that respect, as a "Personal Injury" forensic psychiatric evaluation, this example is not an unusual one, although it does present an extreme example of trauma.

Issues of concern in this type of matter to both plaintiff (and plaintiff's mental health experts) and defense (and defense mental health experts) include the extent to which the traumatic event in question (a rape, in this case) has been the only such incident during a relevant period of time for the victim.

On the other hand, other intervening variables (such as a drug or alcohol problem; a conflicted and abusive marriage or relationship with a partner; a stressful and difficult workplace situation; childhood abuse and trauma; other traumatic experiences such as motor vehicle accidents before and/or after the incident in question; and other such events) may be relevant to the plaintiff's mental state and psychiatric/neuropsychiatric/addiction medicine condition at the time.

In this regard, when such intervening variables may be relevant, a thorough and complete history, buttressed (whether supportive or not) by all potentially available records and materials pertaining to an individual's background and history, should be obtained by the evaluating mental health professional. (These records and materials include medical and psychiatric/psychological diagnostic and treatment records and consultations, employment records, school records, military service records, drug and alcohol treatment records, and any other potentially available such materials. This is the case, clearly, for both criminal and civil forensic mental health evaluations.)

Although Dr. Froyed recognized in her report the bases for the lawsuit in question (i.e., as an alleged deviation from accepted standards of security and safety by a landlord), she did not in this report offer quasi-legal opinions about that deviation. Whereas in professional liability/malpractice actions in which alleged deviations from accepted standards of care of practice are at issue, in this case, such an opinion by a clinical expert (not an expert in building safety and security) would be inappropriate. Dr. Froyed properly focused her evaluation and report on specific forensic mental health issues requested by retaining counsel in this personal injury action.

As with Dr. Fence's criminal report, Dr. Froyed prepared her report as a way chronologically to catalog and review material and testify, if necessary, similar to the way litigating attorneys prepare a trial notebook.

Ultimately, this case was resolved through negotiations and settlement without the necessity for trial or expert testimony by Dr. Froyed. However, retaining defense counsel advised Dr. Froyed prior to the final resolution of this matter that her evaluation and report were instrumental in what defense counsel referred to as "damage control," and in negotiating what defense counsel characterized as a "reasonable settlement."

The straightforward closure that a carefully reasoned and persuasively written opinion can give to a complex report is another pointer of the attorney/expert or court/expert relationship: jargon-free, clear, and convincing writing responsive to the needs of the court or retaining attorney.

What follows is the full forensic expert's report, to give the reader an accurate picture of the final report, as submitted to retaining counsel or to the court.

Full Report

Following up on our telephone discussions and correspondence about the above-referenced matter, and based on the sources of information given below, I am writing you this report of my psychiatric/neuropsychiatric evaluation of Ms. Penelope Jane Holmes in this matter.

This report is provided at your request, and is intended to give you my psychiatric/neuropsychiatric opinion—held with a degree of reasonable medical probability—about Ms. Holmes's present mental state and psychiatric/neuropsychiatric condition and its relationship, if applicable, to her experience of having been sexually assaulted (raped) on October 14, XXXX, in her apartment in Gotham City, Batstate, as described in further detail below.

At this early point in this present evaluation and report, I emphasize that the focus of this present evaluation and report is on Ms. Holmes's *present* psychiatric/neuropsychiatric condition, and is based on the sources of information described below. In this context, I note Ms. Holmes's history of an incident that occurred when she was 9 years old (to be discussed in further detail below), which resulted, among other points, in her feeling of distrust of mental health professionals, a distrust that she describes as having ramifications to the present in terms of her not having sought psychiatric/psychological help or counseling following the October 14, XXXX, incident in question. This and associated issues will be discussed in further detail below.

In this present report, after initially listing and discussing records and materials that I reviewed in connection with this evaluation and report, I will present and discuss Ms. Holmes's background and history as to the time of the October 14, XXXX, incident in question; and as to the time of my interview/examination of her in my office on December 20, XXXX, will present and discuss my psychiatric/neuropsychiatric observations and findings concerning Ms. Holmes from my interview/examination of her; will present and discuss my clinical diagnostic impressions of Ms. Holmes; and will conclude this report (in the section entitled "Summary and Opinions") with a discussion of Ms. Holmes's present psychiatric/neuropsychiatric condition and its relationship, again if applicable, to the October 14, XXXX, incident in question.

For further information and details about Ms. Holmes's background and history; her history up to the time of the October 14, XXXX, incident in question and its aftermath, to the present; and other such aspects of this matter, the reader is referred to applicable records and materials, described below.

The sources of information on which this present evaluation and report are based are as follows:

1. My review of copies of records and materials provided to me by your office in connection with this matter, as follows:

   a. A collection of employment/administrative records and materials pertaining to Ms. Holmes's present employment issues (she is employed with a fashion design firm in Gotham City, Batstate), psychiatric/neuropsychiatric or otherwise, pertaining to the October 14, XXXX, incident in question.

      For information and administrative/employment, payment, and related details contained in this collection, the reader is referred to it.

   b. "Interrogatories" (from defense to plaintiff) and "Answers to Interrogatories" (from plaintiff to defense) in this matter, dated July 10, XXXX, and undated, respectively. The interrogatories, for present purposes, are requesting a "Detailed description of injury or condition claimed to be permanent together with all present complaints" (Interrogatory 4), as well as a "Detailed description of nature, extent and duration of any and all injuries" (Interrogatory 3). The answer to Interrogatory 3 indicated that "I had bruises . . . I suffered emotional injuries. I continue to feel pain and discomfort . . . so I believe these injuries are permanent"; and the answer to Interrogatory 4 was as follows: "See prior answer. My present complaints include: I have a feeling of worthlessness . . . I feel dirty . . . I am very depressed and sad. I feel basically hopeless."

Concerning the issue of treatment, Ms. Holmes's answer to Interrogatory 8 ("It's still being treated") addresses that issue: "I may see a therapist but right now I do not feel trust in anyone to do that."

The answer to Interrogatory 2 gave a detailed account of the rape incident in Ms. Holmes's apartment in Gotham City during the early morning hours of October 14, XXXX. The reader is referred to that answer for further information and details.

c. A collection of medical records and materials from Dr. Goodwin Bones (orthopedist), including clinical notes as well as a copy of chart entries and progress notes from Ms. Holmes's emergency department evaluation and treatment at the Gotham City Medical Center (GCMC; Gotham City, Batstate). Dr. Bones's notes for present purposes, to my reading, do not specifically discuss Ms. Holmes's sexual assault. However, "GCMC Emergency Department Nurses Notes" do.

The "Multi-Disciplinary Assessment/Progress Notes" (Section 4) evaluation states the following:

> Pt. [patient] tearful, but cooperative in answering questions appropriately. C/O [complains of] sexual assault and brought to ER by GCPD. +[present vaginal penetration] with penis. –anal penetration. –[no] oral contact/sex . . . Pt. stated she tried to wrestle with . . . assailant to "get away," but assailant had gun + and she "feared for her life."
>
> States assailant tied her wrists . . . Pt. states assailant lifted her shirt to expose her breasts, took off her underwear and shorts.

d. A letter from Dr. Bones to Clarence Darrow, III, Esquire (Ms. Holmes's counsel in this matter), undated and forwarded to you by Mr. Darrow in a transmittal letter dated May 31, XXXX. Dr. Bones wrote about Ms. Holmes, saying she "came to my office on November 10, XXXX, for injuries as a result of an incident that had occurred on October 14, XXXX. Firstly, she was in a great deal of mental and emotional distress. I had to approach her with very gentle care because her body was in such a guarded and protective state. . . . She then had to seek other forms of treatment to address her needs. I feel that this incident has given her a real setback which she is slowly recovering from. . . . She came for a total of 14 visits."

e. A collection of criminal/legal/discovery records and materials from the Gotham City Police Department pertaining to the police response and investigation of the rape incident against Ms. Holmes of October 14, XXXX. Records and materials consisted of the Incident Reports from responding officers and other such records and materials.

To my reading, the summary of the incident in question, by Police Officer Theo Roosevelt, is the most detailed, as follows:

> Upon arrival the victim stated as she came out of her kitchen into her living room she observed a male with a dark hooded sweat shirt coming out of her bathroom. The actor and the victim began struggling; the actor then forced the victim into the bedroom, tied her hands behind her back, and covered her face with a shirt. When the victim was screaming the actor then retrieved the radio from the kitchen and placed it in the living room on the floor and played the music real loud.

Actor then crawled up on top of the victim, pulled her shirt up kissing her breasts and pulled her panties and shorts down. The victim told the actor she was sick and he better have a condom. He stated, "Oh of course," and she believed he put it on. The actor then inserted his penis into her vagina. After completing the act the actor stated to the victim, "DON'T TELL ANYONE. I KNOW WHERE YOU LIVE. I'M GOING TO KILL YOU." Actor then left through the bedroom apartment window.

For further information contained in police reports and related records and materials contained in this collection, the reader is referred to it.

f. A psychiatric evaluation report and C.V. for Marcus Welby, Jr., MD, in this matter, indicating that Ms. Holmes had been seen in consultation on July 1, XXXX. These two materials were sent under a transmittal letter to you from Mr. Darrow, dated August 10, XXXX.

In his report, Dr. Welby first noted that the purpose of the evaluation was "to evaluate her [Ms. Holmes's] psychiatric condition," and he next listed the five sets of records and materials that he had reviewed in connection with his evaluation. The "Description of Injury" section of the report, to my reading, was lengthy, and elaborated on summaries given, for example, in the police reports noted above. The reader is referred to those sections of Dr. Welby's report for details.

After discussing the events in the October 14, XXXX, incident in question of her subsequent evaluation at the GCMC, Dr. Welby wrote, "In the late morning, Ms. Holmes was able to leave the hospital. She and Vincent were escorted by a police detective to the SAVA Unit at the local precinct house in order for the incident to be recorded. She was again expected to describe the details of the rape, which was overwhelming. After approximately two hours, she could no longer deal with the stress. She became very angry at this point, so the police ended their query and drove Ms. Holmes and Vincent home. When she arrived at her apartment, Ms. Holmes found that most of the surfaces were covered with black fingerprint powder, and that the door to the apartment was taped . . . She went to visit with her childhood friend, who lives in northern Batstate, for a few weeks. Upon her return, she moved to another apartment. Though she would have preferred moving to another apartment complex, she and Vincent were not able to afford this type of a move."

Next in the report, Dr. Welby described Ms. Holmes's symptomatic responses to the incident in question from a psychiatric perspective, noting such symptomatology consistent with posttraumatic stress disorder (PTSD) as Ms. Holmes "continues to persistently reexperience the rape via recurrent and intrusive distressing recollections of the rape. She frequently experiences flashbacks of the rape, and continues to have illusions of 'shadows' of men in her apartment. . . . Numbing of general responsiveness is manifested via anhedonia, feelings of detachment and estrangement from others, a restricted range of affect, and a sense that life will encompass multiple strategies . . . a substantial decrease in appetites accompanied by gastrointestinal distress and weight loss, an extreme delay in sleep onset, which finally occurred when the sun began to rise, accompanied by sleeping into the early afternoon, nonrestorative sleep, psychomotor retardation, a sense of immobilization ... excessive anxiety and worry about a number of issues that typically relate to trust, safety, vulnerability, and the future ... panic attacks, which she continues to experience approximately twice a week. These attacks began when Ms. Holmes returned to work. The anticipatory anxiety regarding her ability to function effectively and cope with her sense of vulnerability may have been the precipitating factor for most of the attacks. Anticipatory anxiety for future attacks, and avoidant behavior secondary to the attacks, has not developed."

On Mental Status Examination, Dr. Welby noted that "it took time for Ms. Holmes to begin speaking about the rape, due to the intensity of her distress regarding its recollection. Mood was clearly despondent. Affect was consistent with mood, with intermittent tearfulness noted. When discussing the details of the rape, Ms. Holmes appeared to be experiencing flashbacks, which she acknowledged were occurring. Cognition appeared intact."

Next, in his report, Dr. Welby described Ms. Holmes's account of her own personal and developmental history (also discussed below). For present purposes, comparing Ms. Holmes's description of herself before and after the incident in question, Dr. Welby wrote that "Ms. Holmes described herself, prior to the rape, as a physically and socially active woman, who enjoyed her work, her home, and her relationships. She enjoyed movies, dancing, walking through the streets of Gotham City, being with friends, writing poetry, and attending a writer's group. Her desire to help others led her to volunteer with a group for foreign students. . . . Ms. Holmes has no personal history of prior psychiatric illness or intervention, nor a family history for psychiatric illness. She did not serve in the military. She has not been involved in prior litigations. . . . After the rape, she went into a 'black hole,' 'withdrawing into a cell' and feeling unable to bring herself back to life. She describes that every day was tremendously painful, and that her sense of self was broken. Feeling terrified of being alone, she pleaded with Vincent to resign from work and stay home with her to protect her, which he did not do. Vincent continued to work. She began to irrationally blame him for not being at home when the intruder broke in and, therefore, not being able to prevent the rape. She then developed a fear that Vincent would not be available when she needed him the most, which precipitated unrealistic rage, causing her to end their relationship multiple times ...

"Prior to the rape, Ms. Holmes described that she and Vincent had wonderful sexual intimacies. She was proud of her body and comfortable with her sexuality. She felt free, and very much enjoyed lovemaking with Vincent. After she was raped, it took one year before Ms. Holmes was willing to be sexually intimate. Her present sexual intimacies now occur approximately once per month, and no longer feel the same. She states, 'I'm no longer the same person.'"

Subsequently, "Ms. Holmes was informed that the rapist was apprehended. The semen left on her sheet provided the deoxyribonucleic acid (DNA) evidence to track him down. Ms. Holmes felt empowered by having realized at the time of the rape that this would be the clue to his identity and apprehension. She also felt a sense of justice. Though she initially felt a sense of relief that he could no longer kill her, this did not have any impact on her extreme sense of fear and vulnerability."

In terms of employment, Dr. Welby wrote, "Ms. Holmes realized that it was unhealthy for her to be isolated and dysfunctional, although she felt too vulnerable and inadequate after the rape to resume her employment. Ms. Holmes finds she's very forgetful, that her mind will go blank and that she no longer can register information as she did before. Though previously she had been dynamic in problem solving, she now feels overwhelmed. Her sense of inadequacy is pervasive, as is her sadness. Ms. Holmes relates that luckily, her co-workers and supervisors have been very supportive of her. A co-worker gave her a car, but she was too frightened to drive, due to her insecurities, and feared that she would get into a fatal accident. Instead, she commutes by public transportation . . . which is a long trip."

In terms of diagnostic considerations, Dr. Welby gave the following using the nosology and format of the *DSM-IV-TR* (also described below):

Axis I (Posttraumatic Stress Disorder):

Major depressive disorder, single episode severe, without psychotic features.

Axis II

No diagnosis.

Axis III

No general medical condition.

Axis IV (Psychosocial and Environmental Stressors):

Unsafe home environment in which rape occurred, causing severe depression, immobilization, and interpersonal conflict.

Axis V (Global Assessment Functioning):

Score of 52.

Finally, in terms of "Treatment Recommendations," Dr. Welby recommended "a combination of pharmacotherapy and psychotherapy for Ms. Holmes's treatment." She also noted that, "Unfortunately, due to this sense of vulnerability and feared victimization, Ms. Holmes has not felt able to commit to psychiatric treatment for fear if she were to open herself to a therapeutic process, it would leave her vulnerable to the physician." (As discussed in further detail below, when Ms. Holmes related her history to me she indicated her sense of concern about a repeat betrayal by a treating psychiatrist, as she had previously experienced when she was 9 years old, and as also discussed above.)

Dr. Welby's "Impression" in this report was that "aforementioned psychiatric illnesses are directly related to and caused by the rape that occurred on October 14, XXXX. Due to the intensity of the trauma, and the severity of the subsequent psychiatric deterioration, permanent psychiatric sequelae are to be expected."

g. A copy of the transcript of Ms. Holmes's deposition in this matter, taken on July 14, XXXX.

To my reading, the content of this deposition reiterates and enlarges on a number of points made in other records and materials (such as police reports, GCMC emergency department evaluation notes for Ms. Holmes, and other such documentation).

For present purposes, in terms of her psychiatric/neuropsychiatric condition and its relationship to the rape incident, and subsequent treatment, Ms. Holmes indicated that she had contacted a crisis hotline following the rape and had spoken with individuals on that hotline twice, and that she had seen Dr. Welby for an evaluation, but was not involved in any psychiatric treatment following the incident in question. She also indicated that when she was 9 years old, she had "an experience in school a long time ago" that influenced her decision not to seek psychiatric treatment following the rape incident in question.

Ms. Holmes testified in her deposition that she "was like 9 years old and we had a psychologist at school and I shared some very private things with her and she went and told the principal and I was expelled from school. . . . I was living with my great aunt and two neighbors came on to me and were trying to seduce me every night late at night after everybody went to sleep, and although there was never a sexual interaction, there was a very sexual nature to it and I was—I felt totally trapped and I went to look for help to the psychologist of the school. The psychologist told the principal about what I shared with her, which I thought was confidential, and out of that, I was expelled from school, I was humiliated, my mother was humiliated, my family was—I was stuck for at least more than seven months at home totally ashamed and trapped out of trying to reach for help and being, like, open and vulnerable with authority about the issue and totally being betrayed and that's why I haven't been able to reach psychological help because even though I know I need it and even though I must do it, I can't bring myself to do it, so that's why I keep postponing and I keep putting it off to call professional help regarding this issue."

In terms of the consequences of the October 14, XXXX, rape incident in question, Ms. Holmes also testified in her deposition that "I totally lost my senses of self, my self-confidence, my self-esteem, I feel broken and fragmented, I feel unsafe in general, I don't have certainty about the things that I used to be certain about, like my career and my emotional life. My boyfriend . . . is impacted by this incident. . . . Because there is a part of me that blames him for not being there when this happened, as much as I've tried to let go of that and be rational about it that he has nothing to do with it, I keep coming back to that and feeling unprotected with him and it leaves me very uncertain about my future with him. . . . I feel paranoid and I was very—before the incident, I was very free to be outside with people and now I feel that I'm always looking who's around me and feeling like anybody could harm me, which it was not like before that. . . . In my job now, I am noticing that my memory is really bad now. I'm not as sharp as I used to be, and just little, basic simple tasks, and that accompanied by a feeling of inadequacy, not being capable and just feeling ugly. . . . Embarrassed, I feel embarrassed and guilty and ashamed also. . . . I had questions about my career, I was—but no, than that no . . . whether I chose the right thing, whether I would be doing that for the rest of my life or not, those kinds of questions . . . ."

Ms. Holmes also commented in her deposition that in terms of her current status, "Things have gotten better. I'm spending more time with friends, I'm forcing myself to be with people and reach family members that I haven't in a long time so that's been helping me . . . crying? . . . know I am eating better . . . I had diarrhea for a month after the incident and everything that I ate, I vomited, I felt so sick . . . at least 20 pounds . . . [weight loss] . . . Yeah [her weight returned] . . . ."

In terms of additional consequences of the incident in question, Ms. Holmes ended: "Sexually. I am not the same person sexually as I was before . . . not as frequent and also, I'm very suppressed now, where I was not before . . . we've [she and Vincent] been broken up since December on and off a couple of times and finally it happened like three weeks ago. . . . I don't go out as much. I used to go dancing late at night, I used to—once I went camping by myself. I could not dare to do that now. I am always afraid now and I wasn't before. . . . Socially, I was never awkward and I was very social before and now I'm very self-conscious when I'm with people, like, I—I feel that I had this big secret that I am imprisoned by and I feel that I am less than everybody else."

For further information and details contained in this deposition transcript, the reader is referred to it.

2. My psychiatric/neuropsychiatric/addiction medicine interview/examination of Ms. Penelope Holmes in my office on November 30, XXXX, which interview/examination included the administration and subsequent scoring and interpretation of a series of standardized and nonstandardized psychological, chemical dependency, and related tests and inventories, as described below;

3. As part of my psychiatric/neuropsychiatric interview/examination of Ms. Holmes, the administration and subsequent scoring and interpretation of a series of standardized and nonstandardized psychological, chemical dependency, and related tests and inventories, as follows:

   a. The Minnesota Multiphasic Personality Inventory, 2nd Edition, or MMPI-2;

b. The Millon Clinical Multiaxial Inventory, 3rd edition, or MCMI-III;
c. The Beck Depression Inventory, 2nd edition, or BDI-II;
d. The Addiction Assessment (nonstandardized) Questionnaire;
e. The Michigan Alcohol Screening Test, or MAST;
f. The Drug Abuse Screening Test, or DAST;
g. The Alcohol Use Disorders Identification Test, or AUDIT;
h. The Mini-Mental State Examination, or MMSE;
i. The Cognitive Capacity Screening Examination, or CCSE; and
j. The Past Medical History (nonstandardized) Questionnaire; and

4. My knowledge, background, training, and experience in psychiatry and neuropsychiatry, addiction medicine, and forensic psychiatry, and—for present purposes—my work and experience in occupational psychiatry.

History

Ms. Penelope (Penny) Jane Holmes is a 26-year-old (DOB: January 26, XXXX) single (never married; Ms. Holmes has a boyfriend, Vincent, West, CPA, age 32, whom she has been dating since August) white female, currently living in a rented private home in Gotham City, where the rape in question occurred on October 14, XXXX.

Ms. Holmes described a psychologically traumatic event when she was 9 years old (see above), which she said resulted in her distrust of psychologists and therapists for a period of time, but not in permanent psychological consequences of sequelae.

Ms. Holmes has been employed with a fashion design firm in Gotham City, a position that she had held for several years after her graduation from the University of Greenstate, where she majored in art and art history. Ms. Holmes had been born and raised in rural and suburban Greenstate, and had never ventured outside that state for longer than one week until she relocated to Gotham City "to try something new" (her words). In addition to her work with the design firm, Ms. Holmes also was employed part-time at an upscale restaurant "to make ends meet" (her words).

In terms of her own personal and psychosocial background and history, Ms. Holmes is an only child, born and raised in Greenstate in what she described as a "very happy" childhood. Both of Ms. Holmes's parents, Sherwood Holmes and Jane Holmes, died at the ages of 55 and 53, respectively, in XXXX, when Ms. Holmes was in her senior year at college. To the best of her knowledge, both of Ms. Holmes's parents were healthy, and she herself was not aware of any family history of serious medical, psychiatric, or related such problems, even in her elderly grandparents and extended family.

Ms. Holmes described her childhood, adolescence, and young adult years as "very happy" ones, in which she enjoyed college, did well academically, was popular, and enjoyed a number of social and extracurricular activities. While in college and for a period of time before meeting Vincent West, her present boyfriend, Ms. Holmes had several intimate heterosexual relationships. She then met Vincent at a business lunch, and they started dating immediately and exclusively, but not living together (in that regard, Ms. Holmes described that her "independence is very important to me").

With the above background and history, Ms. Holmes's account to me (during my interview/examination of her)—an account that may be compared with others, described above and elsewhere in records and materials available for review—about the rape incident of October 14, XXXX, was as follows:

Vincent was working late, we went to a movie, and I took the subway home, by 1:00 A.M. I opened the door, it was hot. I opened the windows, wide open, to the bathroom, and kitchen. I changed clothes to light clothes, and started to wash dishes. I got wrapped up, did cleaning. I had a bag of garbage. I looked at the clock, 3:00 A.M. I was in the kitchen the entire time. I grabbed garbage and saw a shadow go from the bedroom to the bathroom. I thought it was Vincent. It had to be.

I started toward the door. A man jumped me from the back, and I started screaming. He covered my head with something. I was on the floor struggling, wrestling. "This is not going to happen to me." I couldn't turn over. He tried to asphyxiate me, strangle me, then I stopped. Then I said, "Why are you killing me?" He stopped, and I tried to wrestle. No go. His body is on top of me, torso and head. He took out a gun, I thought my life was in danger. I said, "Don't hurt me." He said, "If you do anything, I'll kill you."

Tied my hands behind my back, stood me up, walked me into the bedroom, sat me on my bed against the wall. I asked him, begged, just go. I tried to convince him there was nothing there. He said, "Where is the money?" It was a stupid apartment to break into. How old are you? "Early twenties." "You don't have to do this." He went into the kitchen when he put me onto the bed, got a boom-box from the kitchen to drown out my screams. Then he comes close, said, "I came here to take something." He kissed my neck. I knew he'd rape me. I screamed. He undressed me, my skirt, kissed my breasts, forced me, I begged him, fought, he raped me. I don't remember if I fought right then. I remembered he's untied me, waited five minutes. He threw my cell phone on the bed. I called 911 on the cell, was told not to clean or shower. Went to the window, he was gone, he'd untied me then. I didn't want to tell Vincent, not to trouble us.

The police came, questioned me in the kitchen. To the hospital, in an ambulance, I was a mess, crying, confused. I told the female ambulance attendant not to tell Vincent, she said I shouldn't go through this alone. She called him, he arrived a few hours later. A crisis protocol for him, too. A female detective drove me to the apartment, I showered, then slept through the afternoon. Vincent stayed there for two nights. There was a trace of DNA on the sheets, they eventually found the perpetrator. I was happy, no stalking, he said he'd kill me if I told anybody.

After that, by her account, Ms. Holmes remained out of work for an extended period of time, indicating that, "I couldn't go back to my job, felt inadequate, couldn't leave the apartment much, felt horrible. I forced myself monthly to send a resume on the Internet. I stayed in the apartment two or three months."

Several months after the rape incident in question, Ms. Holmes was able to return to both of her previous jobs ("My bosses were very understanding and sympathetic. They were both women"). She described her necessary ADLs [Activities of Daily Living] as getting up early in the morning, showering and dressing and preparing her morning coffee, commuting to her principal job by subway, putting in a full day of work from about 8:00 A.M. to about 5:00 A.M., and feeling "better since I began to work again, less of a sense of inadequacy . . . simple tasks take a long time, I sometimes feel paranoid about work . . . get home in about two hours, with Vincent, shower, cook, check my email, go to bed after the 11:00 P.M. news. Noises bother me, sex with Vincent still bothers me."

In terms of psychiatric symptomatology that Ms. Holmes attributes to the rape incident in question, she told me during my interview/examination of her that "concentration is down, like I'm another person. I cry easily, there's sadness and disbelief. I pull out my hair, have moments of madness, sex is still a problem with Vincent, used to be every day. We talk about moving in together and getting married and getting a place together. I haven't missed work, but I daydream at work in the design business, not waitressing."

Ms. Holmes's reasons for initiating the civil lawsuit in this matter, in the context of its relationship to her present psychiatric condition, she told me that she had made that decision "immediately, within the week. Before the incident, I knew there were break-ins, problems with security and heat. It's not right. I don't want that to happen to anybody else. I saw ads for attorneys, and I called them."

Concerning Ms. Holmes's "Three Wishes" (an informal psychological projective technique), she told me that they were to "erase my memory and be as innocent as I once was, feel happy, satisfied, fulfilled . . . make up my mind about Vincent."

Finally, Ms. Holmes's rating of herself (on a scale of 0 to 10, in which 0 represents the worst she has ever felt, and the worst she has ever functioned, and 10 represents the best she has ever felt and the best she has ever functioned), Ms. Holmes gave various estimates for various important periods of her life. For example, she rated herself at 8 on the scale during her childhood and adolescence (not identifying very high or very low points during those years); 9 during her years as a student at the University of Vermont; 9 at obtaining her work in fashion design; 4 as she realized that she needed an extra job to "make ends meet" (see above); 8 at meeting and dating Vincent; 0 at the time of the rape incident in question; 6 currently in terms of her relationship with Vincent; and 5 as of the time of my interview/examination of her, in an overall sense. Ms. Holmes commented in response to my specific question that she would expect to be "maybe a 7 or 8 out of 10" when the above-referenced matter is resolved and she no longer has to contend with the exercises and activities associated with the case, as reminders to her of the rape incident in question.

Mental Status (Psychiatric) Examination

This revealed a well-developed, well-nourished white female who was casually dressed in a green dress, a light coat, and women's boots, and who was neatly groomed with blonde hair.

I introduced myself to her, ascertained her understanding of the purpose and scope of the interview/examination, and advised her of the likelihood non-confidential nature of the evaluation. She told me this was acceptable to her. We then proceeded with the interview/examination.

Throughout the interview/examination, Ms. Holmes was pleasant and co-operative, and initially shy and reticent. As time went on, however, she appeared to become more comfortable and less inhibited to the interview/examination situation, her range affect increased, and she became more interactive with me. Throughout the interview/examination, in my view, Ms. Holmes was forthcoming, pleasant, and cooperative. Throughout this interview/examination, there was no indication of severe affective disorder or symptomatology (such as severe depression, mania, or suicidality), although Ms. Holmes did speak about a number of sad themes in her life, especially after the October 14, XXXX, rape incident in question. Similarly, there was no indication of thought disorder or psychotic processes or symptomatology (such as hallucinations, delusions, loosening of associations, and so forth) during this interview/examination.

Cognitively, Ms. Holmes was alert and oriented in all parameters (time, person, place, and circumstances of and reasons for this interview/examination, including her awareness that there would be no privacy or confidentiality between us associated with this interview/examination; this last point was acceptable to her), and her completion of the two standardized cognitive screening tests (the MMSE and the CCSE). Both test results were unremarkable and not indicative of severe organicity or cognitive impairment. Ms. Holmes's general discussion was consistent, in my view, with her level of life experience and formal education as a liberal arts college graduate.

Ms. Holmes's responses to the several standardized and nonstandardized psychological, chemical dependency, and related tests and inventories—beginning with the MMPI-2—yielded results that were considered invalid because: "There are indications that the test-taker answered randomly to many of the items without regard to their content. The profile appears invalid since it has not been completed properly. Little to no weight should be granted to the following interpretive information" (as described in the "Test-Taking Behavior" section of the computer-generated "Comprehensive Report" for this test).

On the other hand, the computer-generated "Interpretive Report" for Ms. Holmes's completion of the Millon Clinical Multiaxial Inventory, 3rd edition (MCMI-III) was described in that report as valid, in which "On the basis of the test data, it may be assumed that the patient is experiencing a severe mental disorder." That said, possible diagnoses for this set of results included "Major Depression (recurrent, severe, without psychotic features)," "Posttraumatic Stress Disorder," and "Adjustment Disorder With Mixed Anxiety and Depressed Mood" (as described in the "Possible Diagnoses" section of this report).

Consistent with Ms. Holmes's reported and described history of lack of problems in the area of alcohol and substance abuse, her responses to the several chemical dependency tests and inventories (the Addiction Assessment Questionnaire, the Michigan Alcohol Screening Test [MAST], the Drug Abuse Screening Test [DAST], and the Alcohol Use Disorders Indentification Test [AUDIT]) were all indicative of no problems, past or present, in these areas.

Finally, Ms. Holmes's completion of the "Past Medical History" questionnaire indicated an individual in generally good health, not presently (or in the past) taking psychotropic medications or involved in psychiatric treatment, and without a prior history of psychiatric or other major medical problems.

In Ms. Holmes's completion of the "Diagnostic Criteria for PTSD" as presented in the *DSM-IV-TR*, she did not endorse either of the two "A" Diagnostic Criteria, although she did endorse them in her discussion of the October 14, XXXX, rape incident in question, during my interview/examination of her. These two criteria require that, "The person has been exposed to a traumatic event in which both of the following were present: (1) The person experienced, witnessed, or was confronted with an event or events that involved actual or threatened death or serious injury, or a threat to the physical integrity of self or others . . . (2) The person's responses involved intense fear, helplessness, or horror." In terms of Ms. Holmes's responses to other symptomatology in these diagnostic criteria, she endorsed fewer currently than had been the case within six months of the incident itself.

Clinical Diagnostic Impressions

In keeping with the current diagnostic nomenclature and format of the *Diagnostic and Statistical Manual of Mental Disorders, Fourth Edition, Text Revision* (2000), of the American Psychiatric Association, clinical diagnostic impressions for Ms. Holmes can be presented as follows:

Axis I (Clinical Disorders):

1. Major depression, single episode, recurrent, without psychotic features.
2. Posttraumatic stress disorder, chronic.

Axis II (Personality Disorders):

No diagnosis.

Axis III ("General Medical Conditions"):

Ms. Holmes appears to be in generally good medical condition, without indications of active, acute, chronic, or ongoing medical problems or conditions requiring medical attention or treatment.

In this context, however, I note Ms. Holmes's stating a need for psychiatric treatment for problems and symptomatology associated with the October 14, XXXX, rape incident in question, despite her unwillingness to be involved in such treatment.

Axis IV (Psychosocial and Environmental Problems):

As a practical clinical matter, Ms. Holmes's main present "Psychosocial and Environmental Problems" relate to symptomatology associated with the October 14, XXXX, rape incident in question, and its aftermath. Otherwise, by her account, she has a supportive relationship with a boyfriend, is gainfully employed and hardworking, has adequate housing, has resumed sexual activities with her boyfriend (although, by her account, not to the pre-rape incident level), and has a sufficient educational background to employ her in professional work that she finds enjoyable and fulfilling, if not sufficiently financially rewarding.

These and "Problems related to interactions with the legal system," specifically referring to exercises and activities associated with the above-referenced lawsuit and its periodic reminders and associations to her of the October 14, XXXX, rape incident in question, constitute, in my view, Ms. Holmes's main "Environmental and Psychosocial Problems" at this point. In that regard, Ms. Holmes herself estimated that her "self-rating" (see above) will be higher for her once the above-referenced lawsuit has been resolved.

Axis V (Global Assessment of Functioning [GAF]):

A GAF Scale score of 60–70 signifying mild-to-moderate impairment and symptomatology, in my opinion, applies here.

Summary and Opinions

Ms. Penelope Jane Holmes is a 26-year-old (DOB: January 26, XXXX) white female, educated and trained in areas of fashion and design, currently employed in that capacity with a firm in Gotham City, Batstate, and currently involved with her boyfriend, "Vincent," with whom she has had what she described as an on-and-off relationship since they first started dating in May of XXXX.

With that background, Ms. Holmes was involved in the rape episode at her apartment in Gotham City during the early morning hours of October 14, XXXX, as described above and elsewhere in records and materials available for review in this matter. Following that incident, Ms. Holmes was evaluated on an emergency basis at the GCMC, and on occasions after that, made calls to a local hotline for counseling and support. She has not been involved in psychiatric treatment since that time, notwithstanding her acknowledgment that such treatment would be clinically indicated for her. She also remained out of work for an extended period of time after the incident in question, eventually returning to her present job.

With this background and history, Ms. Holmes instituted the above-referenced lawsuit against her apartment owners. In the context of that lawsuit, your office arranged for this present second opinion (my characterization, a second opinion to that of Dr. Marcus Welby, described above) to explore the issue of Ms. Holmes's present psychiatric/neuropsychiatric condition and its relationship, if so, to her rape experience of October 14, XXXX.

The sources of information on which this present evaluation and report are based; Ms. Holmes's background and history leading up to the time of the rape incident in question; and then to the time of my interview/examination of her in this matter; my psychiatric/neuropsychiatric observations and findings concerning Ms. Holmes; and my clinical diagnostic impressions of Ms. Holmes are all as described above and elsewhere in records and materials available for review in this matter. That information will not be repeated in this section of this report.

Ms. Holmes's present psychiatric/neuropsychiatric condition, with associated diagnoses and levels of functioning, is as described above. While I do not significantly disagree, to my reading, with Dr. Welby's formulation of Ms. Holmes's present situation, I note that in the context of her life in general,

Ms. Holmes's present self-rating (see above) is not very much different from self-ratings at other various points in her life (some of which have been psychologically traumatic for her); and that her own estimate of this rating as well as her endorsement of fewer symptoms in the Diagnostic Criteria of PTSD (since the time of the incident itself) shows improvement and amelioration in her clinical condition since the time of the incident itself. In that sense, as a "survivor" (my word; see above), Ms. Holmes may be considered to have "survived" the immediate and longer-term trauma of the October 14, XXXX, rape incident at issue.

In that vein, I note Dr. Welby's recommendation for psychotherapy and pharmacotherapy for Ms. Holmes. Ms. Holmes herself agreed that such treatment would be desirable for her. However, despite the advisability of such treatment for her, Ms. Holmes has managed to do as well as she has been doing—personally, professionally, socially, and with her boyfriend—without such help. This underscores her being a survivor, in my view. As contemplated by Dr. Welby, effective psychiatric treatment would likely help with Ms. Holmes's self-esteem, work-related symptomatology (e.g., her perception of memory problems), and her overall well-being: I agree that Ms. Holmes would be well advised to become involved in such treatment, but also note her current good functioning without such treatment.

Putting these various points together, it is my psychiatric/neuropsychiatric opinion—held with a degree of reasonable medical probability—that while Ms. Penelope Jane Holmes has experienced PTSD and other psychiatric problems as a result of the rape incident of October 14, XXXX, her response to that incident has been influenced and informed by her prior experience (referring, for example, to Ms. Holmes's self-ratings at various points in her life, both before and after the October 14, XXXX, incident in question); that notwithstanding that incident and its aftermath, Ms. Holmes has been able to continue her relationship with her boyfriend, Vincent, and to obtain work and thereby become independent in her day-to-day functioning again; that Ms. Holmes has been able to achieve these gains without psychiatric treatment and/or psychopharmacotherapy; and that, in sum, Ms. Holmes's status as a survivor (see above) has permitted her to do as well as she has been able to do, despite the rape incident itself and her lack of specific treatment or therapy after the incident to address the consequences and sequelae of that incident.

Finally, in the context of this present evaluation and report, I reiterate Ms. Holmes's perception that the stresses and reminders of exercises and activities associated with the litigation in this matter, which remind her and reinforce her feelings about the incident itself, once concluded, will permit her to move on and to increase her perception (i.e., her self-rating) in terms of her overall level of functioning and happiness.

The referenced individual was examined with reference to specific issues emanating from the original situation, in accordance with the restrictive rules concerning an independent medical examination. It is, therefore, understood that no treatment was given or suggested and that no doctor/patient relationship exists.

I aver that the information contained in this document was prepared by the undersigned and is the work of the undersigned. It is true to the best of my knowledge and information and has not been modified by anyone other than the undersigned.

Please advise me if you have questions about this present evaluation and report, or if you anticipate requiring additional services from me in connection with this matter.

Thank you very much.

Selma J. Froyed, MD

Board of Employment Commissioners (BEC) v. Paul Strong, et al., and *Charlene Boyle v. Paul Strong, et al.*

Case Overview: Sexual Harassment in the Workplace

This is a lawsuit brought by a former employee, Charlene Boyle. The attorney representing the plaintiff, Boyle, retained the services of a psychiatrist, Steven L. Meade, MD, MS, to evaluate the plaintiff's mental condition and related damages allegedly caused by workplace harassment. Dr. Meade's report follows.

The Report

> Forensic mental health evaluations in employment law matters illustrate very well the distinction between liability (*not* addressed in these evaluations) and damages (the purpose and focus of these evaluations) in civil matters, as is also the case in forensic mental health evaluations in personal injury matters (such as *Holmes v. Moriarty Real Estate, et al.,* the first of these four civil case evaluation reports). A clear statement early in the report (occurring in the first paragraph, in this report) makes that important distinction clear.

At your request, and based on the sources of information given below, I am writing you this report of my psychiatric evaluation of Ms. Charlene Boyle in order to assess Ms. Boyle's present clinical psychiatric/neuropsychiatric/addiction medicine condition and its relationship, if applicable, to her period of alleged sexual harassment by Mr. Paul Strong. This alleged harassment occurred in the context of her employment with the Strong Battery Company from February XXXX (when the alleged harassment by Mr. Strong began) to the fall of XXXX (when Ms. Boyle left her position with Strong).

In this context, I emphasize at this early point in the report, that this evaluation and report are intended to address the issue of psychiatric and psychological issues, if applicable, with Ms. Boyle, pertaining to effects on her of her alleged harassment by Mr. Strong. This evaluation and report are *not* intended to address the issue of whether, in fact, the harassment actually took place. An opinion about that issue would be administrative/legal (employment law), and not within the scope of this present clinically oriented report.

> By making the point early in the report that the evaluation and report are clinical in nature, the writer establishes at the outset that this report addresses the damages (psychiatric/neuropsychiatric/addiction medicine) issue, if applicable, and not the liability issue.

Since Ms. Boyle's past history; the history of her alleged harassment by Mr. Strong; her history since her having left Strong Battery Company; her family history; and other such aspects and elements of this matter are detailed in the extensive and voluminous records and materials available for review in connection with this matter, I will not reiterate details contained in these other records and materials in this report.

Rather, after briefly reviewing Ms. Boyle's background and history; the history of her period of alleged sexual harassment by Mr. Strong; her history and situation since that period of time; her family history; and so forth, I will focus on my present neuropsychiatric findings and impressions of Ms. Boyle. I will conclude this report with a description of that neuropsychiatric condition and my professional opinion—held with a degree of reasonable medical probability—of the relationship, if applicable, between Ms. Boyle's present situation and her period of alleged sexual harassment by Mr. Strong (February XXXX to the fall of XXXX).

For further details about these various aspects of Ms. Boyle's situation, as just described, please refer to the records and materials described below.

> As with most of the reports in this book—both criminal and civil—a cataloging, listing, and summarizing of legal and clinical records reviewed in the preparation of this report enables the evaluator to reread and learn the contents of the records and materials, and also enables the evaluator to construct a document parallel to the attorney's trial notebook. This, in turn, promotes efficient and responsive communication between the forensic evaluator and retaining counsel/court, both important elements, or pointers (Chapter 1) in the attorney/expert and court/expert process.

The sources of information on which this evaluation and report are based are as follows:

1. My review of extensive and voluminous legal, medical, therapy, and related records and materials pertaining to this matter, as described below. In view of the voluminous and varied nature of these records and materials, rather than listing and describing each of them, I will refer at this point in this report to them generally, incorporating their substance later in the "History" section of this report.

In a general sense, records reviewed consisted of legal materials (e.g., Ms. Boyle's original BEC complaints; correspondence pertaining to this matter; various Certifications and BEC "Determinations" [made by Alfred Towle, Area Director in May XXXX, determining that there was "cause to believe" that Ms. Boyle was sexually harassed as charged] and other such records and materials); clinical and therapy records, notes, and materials (from Dr. Richard Truman, including an affidavit by Dr. Truman pertaining to this [Dr. Truman has been Ms. Boyle's treating psychologist, from October XXXX to the present]; from Dr. Merle Brown, who performed a psychological evaluation on Ms. Boyle, which included evaluation notes, two [2] reports of November 14, XXXX, and January 11, XXXX, and a videotape of Dr. Brown's first evaluation session; from Dr. Melvin Rotha, who did a disability evaluation for the State Department of Labor, dated October 20, XXXX; the Social Security Administration records used to determine Ms. Boyle's eligibility for Social Security Benefits; from Dr. Lorena Hickey, who did an adjunctive psychological evaluation and testing in connection with this evaluation and report, emphasizing evaluation of dissociative aspects of Ms. Boyle; from Dr. John Gregory [psychiatrist; June 12, XXXX]; and from other physicians and health service providers affiliated with the Trinity Health Plan, Ms. Boyle's HMO at the time [XXXX] whom she saw for evaluation and treatment of anxiety symptomatology); deposition transcripts (for the depositions of Ms. Boyle herself, Ms. Boyle's mother, Prudence Boyle, and of her two sisters, Jean Boyle, and Barbara Boyle, all taken in May XXXX); notes and materials from Ms. Charlene Boyle herself (including her "The Journal" from September XXXX through December XXXX; a family diary of mental illness and death, dated June 9, XXXX, and a "Lifestyle Analysis," dated May 12, XXXX, both prepared for a college course); correspondence from U.S. Representative Simon Holmby's office to Ms. Boyle pertaining to her complaints of sexual harassment; affidavits by Ms. Boyle concerning alleged acts of sexual harassment by Mr. Strong and physical and sexual abuse by her ex-husband; and Wallace College transcripts for Ms. Boyle;

2. My two psychiatric interviews/examinations of Ms. Boyle in my office on September 14, XXXX, and October 9, XXXX, respectively. These interviews/examinations included, in part, a clinical interview/examination by Dr. Lorena Hickey, who also administered a series of psychological tests and inventories having to do, in large part, with dissociative phenomena and related aspects of Ms. Boyle's situation;

3. As part of my interviews/examinations of Ms. Boyle, the administration and subsequent scoring and interpretation of a series of standardized and non-standardized psychological, chemical dependency, and related tests and inventories, as follows:

   a. The Minnesota Multiphasic Personality Inventory, 2nd edition, or MMPI-3 (also administered by Dr. Brown);
   b. The Millon Clinical Multiaxial Inventory, 3rd edition, or MCMI-III;
   c. The Beck Depression Inventory, 2nd edition, or BDI-II;
   d. The Addiction Assessment (nonstandardized) survey instrument;
   e. The Drug Abuse Screening Test, or DAST;
   f. The Michigan Alcohol Screening Test, or MAST;

g. The Alcohol Use Disorders Identification Test, or AUDIT;

h. The Mini-Mental State Examination, or MMSE;

i. The Cognitive Capacity Screening Examination, or CCSE; and

j. The Past Medical History (nonstandardized) survey instrument; and

4. My knowledge, background, training, and experience in psychiatry and neuropsychiatry, and especially in my work with victims of abuse and trauma.

Unlike in the previous case (*Holmes*), the plaintiff in this matter, Charlene Boyle, had a seriously dysfunctional, abusive, and damaged background and history leading up to her workplace experiences at issue in this employment law matter (alleged sexual harassment). Describing that background and history in detail in the report permits the core forensic mental health issue in this evaluation—Ms. Boyle's present psychiatric condition and its relationship, if so, to her workplace experiences—to be addressed specifically later in the report. The "History" section of this report needs to be detailed, to flow into her work experiences at issue in the case, and to draw a contrast between Ms. Boyle's pre- and post-workplace activities and level of functioning.

History

Ms. Charlene Elizabeth Boyle is a 49-year-old (DOB: January 3, XXXX) divorced white female, living in her private home with her widowed mother, Prudence Boyle (age 73), her daughter, Kathleen Clark (age 24), and her "life partner," Ms. Wanda Elliot (age 52). Ms. Boyle is currently a student in a master's program in speech pathology at Wallace College, with which program she has been affiliated since the fall of XXXX.

Ms. Boyle was born and raised in Bowville, and early in her childhood, her family relocated to Brooklyn. Ms. Boyle's father was a baker, and her mother was a homemaker.

Ms. Boyle is the oldest in a sibship of three sisters, with one sister, Jean Boyle (age 38), divorced from an abusive and violent husband. Jean has two sons and a daughter, all of whom are involved in counseling (through a battered woman's shelter program). Barbara Boyle (age 29, single, and described by Ms. Boyle having "felt she was in an abusive relationship—she solicited drugs and prostitution") is particularly troubled and psychiatrically disturbed at present.

Ms. Boyle described a very dysfunctional, abusive, and upsetting childhood and upbringing, characterized by physical abuse of herself and her sisters by her mother, and by sexual abuse of herself and her sisters both by her father, Dennis Boyle, and subsequently by two of her mother's boyfriends.

Ms. Boyle's childhood was also marked by her father's having left the family when Ms. Boyle was approximately 9 years old, and by his later suicide, committed after a period of over 12 years of no contact with Ms. Boyle or with his family. Ms. Boyle claims that her father had sexually molested and abused her from about age six until he left his family, and that he had also abused and molested her sisters. She related that her mother did not defend her or her sisters against her father's abuse because of her own weakness, but that she, Ms. Boyle herself—because of her having been the oldest daughter by many years—had a responsible role in her family to help take care of her younger sisters.

Two of Ms. Boyle's sisters left home while young teenagers, becoming prostitutes and living on the streets. After her father left the family, Ms. Boyle described having had a "nervous breakdown," necessitating her hospitalization at the Orange County Hospital Center (OCHC) for psychiatric hospitalizations for two several-month periods; these hospitalizations occurred when she was 12 and 13 years old. After that, Ms. Boyle was referred to the Tower Hills residential treatment center, where she remained as a voluntary patient from ages 13 through 17. She described having been a good student and having done well at that center. She also states that her mother began to drink alcohol to excess at that point, subsequently developing an alcohol problem, after her husband (Ms. Boyle's father) had left.

Ms. Boyle also states that her mother began to bring boyfriends to her home after that point. Two of the men reportedly sexually molested Ms. Boyle and/or her sisters, one during the time before Ms. Boyle's first admission to OCHC and another after her transfer to the Tower Hills residential treatment center. Ms. Boyle was frequently in conflict with her mother about these men, and she described her institutionalization at Tower Hills as therapeutic, beneficial, and a relief for her.

At about age 14, Ms. Boyle met Mr. Ken Clark, whom she later married. She became pregnant by him at age 14, while at Tower Hills, and was sent home with recommendations for an abortion. She did have the abortion, which she described as very traumatic, painful, and lonely (she was in labor, left alone for three days for the abortion to be completed, describing that experience as demeaning and horrible). The effects of this abusive situation on her sisters were also profound. Ms. Boyle also related that one of them became pregnant by age 14, one married an abusive man at age 16, and one left home at age 14 to become a prostitute.

After Ms. Boyle completed her program at the Tower Hills, she transferred to a residential halfway house, attended high school, and lived in a supported residential situation until she was 18. She married Mr. Clark during that time, who was sexually, emotionally, physically, and verbally abusive to her, by her description, from the beginning of that marriage. She described, for example, that her ex-husband had raped her, and had played "Russian roulette" (i.e., with a gun) with her. Ms. Boyle regards this period of time of her life as dysfunctional and disturbing for her, requiring that she mature and take on responsibility earlier than she had wanted to, and exposing her to intimate knowledge and experience with abusive men and abusive situations.

Ms. Boyle eventually obtained a GED, and after that, began work in retailing, engaging in that type of work up to and including her six years with Strong Battery Company, from XXXX through XXXX.

The issue of deviant and destructive childhood and adolescent sexuality for Ms. Boyle was emphasized in this section of this report. The author rightfully felt that sexuality and its determinants were central to this evaluation of alleged *sexual* harassment of Ms. Boyle in her workplace.

Following her marriage to Mr. Clark, Ms. Boyle had one child by him (Kathleen Clark, now age 24), and began her career in the photo retailing industry. She described a very difficult and abusive relationship with her husband, and eventually separated from him in XXXX, with her divorce becoming final several years after that. She has had no social/sexual contact with men since then, but has had a committed relationship with her life partner, Wanda, for about the past 10 years. She has lived with Wanda "as lovers" (her words) for about the past 8 years (Ms. Boyle's household at this point consists of herself, Wanda, her mother, and her daughter).

Since Ms. Boyle's separation from her husband, she describes her life as generally stable and personally and professionally satisfactory. This had been the case leading up to the period of time of her alleged sexual harassment by Mr. Paul Strong, as described in this report and elsewhere in available records and materials.

With regard to Ms. Boyle's reported sexual harassment by Mr. Strong, since available records and materials describe this in considerable detail, I will summarize that alleged harassment in this report, and not reiterate those records here.

> **After presenting Ms. Boyle's strangely dysfunctional personal, social, and sexual background, including a period of relative calm after her separation from her abusive husband, the report next focuses on Ms. Boyle's account of her workplace experiences with her former employer during the period of time in question.**

Ms. Boyle described how she had worked at the Strong Battery Company from XXXX through XXXX, and how the first actual incident of harassment occurred in September XXXX. At that point, Ms. Boyle attained the position of sales manager for that company. To that time, Ms. Boyle described enjoying her work and her work environment very much, feeling like "a member of the family," admiring Mr. Strong and believing that Mr. Strong's character and behavior were "impeccable" (her word). Mr. Strong reportedly propositioned Ms. Boyle in August of XXXX, and then put her physically in a position where it was difficult for her to get away from him ("he pushed me up against the wall, body-pressed me, put his hands on my breasts, knee in my groin"). This was upsetting to Ms. Boyle, in that she felt threatened and afraid, as well as worried about jeopardizing her position with Mr. Strong's company because of her refusing his reported advances.

Nothing was said about that incident, and Ms. Boyle gradually felt better about it. As the fall of that year (XXXX) came, she described being hopeful that this situation would pass over. During that time, another incident of reported sexual harassment by Mr. Strong occurred while Ms. Boyle and he were driving back to the office from an outside meeting. During that incident, Mr. Strong reportedly "grabbed my hand—pushed it into his crotch." Shortly thereafter, he reportedly threatened Ms. Boyle with retaliation, after reportedly squeezing her breast during a meeting in his office. Ms. Boyle also described several other similar incidents, in the last of which she told how Mr. Strong reportedly "pushed me against the wall, pulled my hand down toward his penis—out of his pants—exposed himself," then stopped. It was at that point that Ms. Boyle decided that she had to leave the company and also decided that she needed psychiatric/psychological help. (Ms. Boyle's psychiatric treatment history has already been described. In addition to her inpatient and residential treatment, she also was involved in psychotherapy/counseling with a Lucille Ward while she was in her abusive marriage with Mr. Clark.)

> **Here in the report, the author notes that by this time, Ms. Boyle had reached the point at which she felt she could no longer maintain silence and do nothing about the reported incidents of sexual harassment by Mr. Strong. First, she decided to leave the company and seek counseling.**

Ms. Boyle contacted a rape crisis counselor named Roseanne Salvato, who subsequently referred her to Dr. Truman, who first saw her in September XXXX, and who has been treating her on a regular and continuing basis since that time. It was also during that time that Ms. Boyle filed her BEC complaint against Mr. Strong, having withdrawn her initial complaint (out of fear of retaliation, by her description) and having later reinstated it.

Ms. Boyle described that she felt tense and anxious from May XXXX through the end of her employment at the Strong Company, because of fear of repercussions of her refusing Mr. Strong's reported advances, and because of reminders and associations that she had with her prior extensive history of sexual abuse, dysfunctional family relations, and so forth.

Following her leaving the Strong company, Ms. Boyle remained unemployed for a period of time, feeling that she had somehow been blacklisted from further employment in the battery product industry because of her experiences at the Strong Company. She eventually was approved for Social Security Disability (on psychiatric grounds; please refer to Dr. Roth's report and her Social Security records for details).

In the summer of XXXX, Ms. Boyle began a new course of study in speech pathology at Wallace College; her Wallace College transcripts indicate that she is doing well in those studies. She is enthusiastic about those studies, enjoys them, and anticipates a successful career as a speech pathologist. In that sense, her present attitude and approach to life are optimistic and enthusiastic, and she feels that she is a survivor (also noted by Dr. Brown in his report) with a favorable outlook and prognosis in life.

> **Ms. Boyle's evaluator, Dr. Meade, draws a contrast here between Ms. Boyle's present positive life circumstances and her difficult circumstances while an employee of the Strong Company.**

Ms. Boyle has an extensive past medical history as well as her extensive psychiatric history. Without reiterating details previously noted in this report and elsewhere in available records and materials, I note that she has had a number of gynecologic problems, including a ruptured ovarian cyst at age 18, with eventual removal (in XXXX) of the chronically painful ovary. She has had gallbladder and peptic ulcer disease problems in her 20s, and problems with endometriosis and adhesions, and bleeding in her 30s. She had a voluntary abortion from her last pregnancy by Mr. Clark, and also a sterilization procedure (bilateral tubal ligation) in connection with that abortion. Approximately 10 years ago, Ms. Boyle fell and sustained a concussion and skull fracture on the right, with subsequent sensorineural hearing loss on the right; she does not otherwise presently describe any sequelae of that injury. Finally, in May XXXX, Ms. Boyle underwent a partial hysterectomy because of fibroids, which has had the effect of eliminating her dysmenorrhea, and which she regards as beneficial to her.

As described above, the records and materials for this matter are extensive and voluminous. This section of this report represents a summary of information available in this matter and of Ms. Boyle's background and history leading up to the time of my interviews/examinations of her on September 12, XXXX, and October 9, XXXX. For further information and details about Ms. Boyle's background and history, the history of her alleged sexual harassment incidents in connection with her employment with the Strong Company, and other such aspects of this matter, the reader is referred to applicable records and materials as described above and elsewhere in records and materials available for review in this matter.

In a quick and informal self-rating scale, Dr. Meade next describes Ms. Boyle's self-rating at various significant points in her life. This technique gives an overview of Ms. Boyle's present level of functioning—the core area to be addressed in this report—and anticipates Dr. Meade's forensic opinion in this matter, as expressed in the "Summary and Opinions" section.

In terms of Ms. Boyle's self-rating (on a scale of 0–10, in which 0 is the worst she has felt and functioned and 10 is the best), she rated her childhood, overall, as a 2; her years of institutionalization during her teenage years as a 0; her relationship with her ex-husband as 4; the birth of her child as 9; her subsequent relationship with and divorce from her husband as 3; the time from her separation and divorce to her beginning work with the Strong Company as 7; her first several years with that company as 8; her period of alleged sexual harassment with the Strong Company as 4; and her subsequent situation and studies as 9.

Ms. Boyle has previously been involved in counseling, psychiatric treatment, and psychotherapy; she has not been involved in those activities, by her account, for the past three years. She is not currently taking any psychotropic medications for anxiety, depression, or other such symptomatology.

Despite Ms. Boyle's preworkplace and postworkplace experiences, as of the time of her forensic mental health evaluation, Ms. Boyle was doing well psychiatrically, and not presenting significant psychiatric symptomatology or psychopathology, except in terms of her anger and resentment toward her former employer. By describing that clinical presentation and demeanor in this section of the report, Ms. Boyle's lack of clinically significant present damages (psychiatric symptomatology) is emphasized in the context of that issue, and, again, a transition into the "Summary and Opinions" section of the report made easier.

Mental Status (Psychiatric) Examination

I introduced myself to Ms. Boyle, ascertained her understanding of the purpose and scope of the interview/examination, and advised her of the likelihood non-confidential nature of the evaluation. She told me this was acceptable to her. We then proceeded with the interview/examination.

Ms. Boyle presented as a well-developed, well-nourished, medium-height and medium-weight white female who was carefully and casually dressed in a woman's navy suit, white blouse, several gold necklaces, and shoes. Ms. Boyle was formal and superficially pleasant and cooperative throughout the interview/examination, reluctantly discussing her background, history, and experiences with the Strong Company, and not forthcoming or spontaneous, in my view. On several occasions, it was necessary to press Ms. Boyle about particular questions—especially those pertaining to her alleged sexual harassment with the Strong Company—but as a practical matter, she did respond to these questions. Her speech was unremarkable with regard to language, flow, and rhythm.

Throughout the interview/examination, there was no indication of severe affective disorder or symptomatology (such as severe depression, mania, or suicidality), nor was there any indication of thought disorder or psychotic processes or symptomatology (such as hallucinations, delusions, loosening of associations, and so forth).

Cognitively, Ms. Boyle was alert and oriented in all parameters (time, person, place, and circumstances of and reasons for this interview/examination, including its nonconfidential nature, which was acceptable to her), and her responses to the two standardized cognitive screening tests (the MMSE and the CCSE) were unremarkable and not indicative of severe organicity or cognitive impairment.

As discussed in Appendix C, psychological testing can be very useful in evaluations, both in giving details of psychopathology of the evaluee, and in giving levels of severity of psychopathology and symptomatology. This was the case in Ms. Boyle's test results and interpretations.

Ms. Boyle's responses to the several standardized and nonstandardized psychological, chemical dependency, and related tests and inventories gave a "Valid Profile," according to the computer-generated "Interpretive Report" for this test, with the "Profile Severity" section of this test indicating that "On the basis of the test data, it may be assumed that this individual is experiencing either no mental disorder [or] . . . mild mental disorder." That said, "Possible Diagnoses" (described using the nosology and format of the *DSM-IV-TR*, as discussed in further detail below) were "adjustment disorder with mixed anxiety and depression" (on Axis I) and "dependent personality traits," "narcissistic personality features," and "borderline personality features" (on Axis II).

Ms. Boyle's score on the BDI-II did not indicate a clinically significant level of depressive symptomatology during the two-week period of time prior to her taking that test, according to published norms for that text. (In my view, this is an unrealistically low level of endorsed test items. That point will be discussed in further detail below.)

Consistent with Ms. Boyle's reported and described lack of history of past or present chemical dependency problems or treatment, her responses to the several chemical dependency tests and inventories (the Addiction Assessment questionnaire; the MAST; the DAST; and the AUDIT) did not indicate any such problems, past or present.

Ms. Boyle's preexisting (to the period of alleged sexual harassment at The Strong Company) psychiatric and medical history was brought out in her responses to the "Past Medical History" inventory.

Finally, Ms. Boyle's responses to the "Past Medical History" questionnaire confirmed her extensive past medical history as well as her extensive past psychiatric history. As mentioned above, her medical conditions have included a number of gynecological problems, including a ruptured ovarian cyst at age 18, with eventual removal (in XXXX) of the chronically painful ovary; gallbladder and peptic ulcer disease problems in her 20s; problems with endometriosis and adhesions, and bleeding in her 30s; a voluntary abortion from her last pregnancy with her ex-husband and a subsequent sterilization procedure (bilateral tubal ligation) following that abortion; a skull fracture on the right and concussion following a fall in approximately XXXX, with subsequent sensorineural hearing loss on her right (she does not describe any present sequelae of that injury); and in XXXX, a partial hysterectomy because of fibroids, which has resulted in the elimination of her dysmenorrhea. Ms. Boyle's dysfunctional family background and history; her father's sexual abuse of her and her sisters, and his subsequent leaving the family; her sense of responsibility for her younger siblings (as the oldest sibling in her family); her psychiatric hospitalization after her father's leaving the family, and her subsequent three-year psychiatric hospitalization; her mother's promiscuity and her own molestation by her mother's boyfriends; her traumatic relationship and early pregnancy with her (later) husband; her difficult and abusive relationship with her husband and eventual separation and divorce; her subsequent lesbian relationship, which she described as happy and stable; and her subsequent reported sexual harassment with the Strong Company, have all been described above and elsewhere in records and materials available for review in this matter. The reader is referred to those records and materials and earlier sections of this report for further information and details contained in those records and in this report.

Clinical Diagnostic Impressions

In keeping with the current diagnostic nomenclature and format of the *Diagnostic and Statistical Manual of Mental Disorders, Fourth Edition, Text Revision* (2000), or *DSM-IV-TR,* of the American Psychiatric Association, clinical diagnostic impressions for Ms. Boyle can be presented as follows:

In our experience, the various iterations of the *DSM* (currently the *DSM-IV-TR*) present a widely used schema for both clinical and forensic mental health data recording and documentation. We strongly recommend its use in forensic reports.

Axis I (Clinical Disorders):

1. Adjustment disorder with mixed anxiety and depression, chronic.
2. Posttraumatic stress disorder, chronic, from a variety of causes.

Axis II (Personality Disorders):

No diagnosis.

Axis III (General Medical Conditions):

Ms. Boyle's extensive medical history and treatment history have already been described; the reader is referred to applicable earlier sections of this report and other records and materials available for review in this matter for further information and details pertaining to that history. Presently, Ms. Boyle's health is good, without indications of present active, chronic, or ongoing medical problems or conditions requiring active intervention or treatment.

Axis IV (Psychosocial and Environmental Problems):

As a practical clinical matter, Ms. Boyle's main present "Psychosocial and Environmental Problems," in my view, pertain to her "Educational problems" (her new program), "Occupational problems" (her present lawsuit), and her "Economic problems" (her current student status and by virtue of that, unemployed status, with subsequent loss of income). However, in that regard, Ms. Boyle described considerable satisfaction with her present course of study in speech pathology, as well as a present happy and stable life and lifestyle.

Axis V (Global Assessment of Functioning [GAF]):

A GAF Scale score of 70–80 signifying that "if symptoms are present, they are transient and expectable reactions to psychosocial stressors . . . no more than slight impairment in social, occupational, or school functioning . . . [to] Some mild symptoms . . . but generally functioning pretty well, has some meaningful interpersonal relationships," in my opinion, applies here.

The several lines of analysis previously laid out in this report up to its last section ("Summary and Opinions") come to fruition here. The core forensic evaluation questions of "How is Ms. Boyle doing now from a forensic perspective, and how does that relate—if it does—to her workplace experiences at issue?" are answered. This last, most important, section of the report needs to be clear, brief, direct, and forceful, as it should be in all of the reports described in this book.

Summary and Opinions

Ms. Charlene Boyle is a 49-year-old (DOB: January 3, XXXX) divorced white female, living in her private home with her widowed mother, Prudence Boyle (age 73), her daughter, Kathleen Clark (age 24), and her "life partner," Ms. Wanda Elliot. Ms. Boyle is currently a student in a master's program in speech pathology at Wallace University, with which program she has been affiliated since the fall of XXXX.

Ms. Boyle described having been involved in a difficult, dysfunctional, and unhappy childhood. She is oldest in a sibship of three sisters, all of whom have had personal, psychosocial, and dysfunctional difficulties during their lives, including her next-oldest sister, who is currently involved in an abusive relationship with a man who "has been a drunk for a long time" (Ms. Boyle's words).

As described above and elsewhere in records and materials available for review in this matter, Ms. Boyle's dysfunctional childhood, adolescence, and adulthood included psychiatric hospitalizations and institutionalizations of her for extended periods of time, her father's having left the family when she was about 9 years old, and his subsequent suicide after many years of no contact with him. Ms. Boyle described herself as having felt responsible for raising her sisters, with her ineffective mother (Ms. Boyle, as mentioned, was the oldest), which problems were subsequently compounded by her early marriage to her former husband. That relationship was also abusive, difficult, and dysfunctional, and after the birth of her children, Ms. Boyle separated and then divorced from her husband. Her life had been somewhat calmer and more stable since that time, leading up to her allegations of sexual harassment by Mr. Paul Strong in her work as sales manager with the Strong Battery Company from XXXX to XXXX.

Leading up to this point in the report, the author summarizes and emphasizes Ms. Boyle's dysfunctional background and history leading up to her employment with the Strong Company.

Ms. Boyle stated that in the last several years of her work with that company—which she had described as a family-oriented company in which she had initially felt comfortable—Mr. Strong reportedly propositioned her in June of XXXX, and at one point, put her physically in a position where it was difficult for her to get away from him ("he pushed me up against the wall, body-pressed me, put his hands on my breasts, knee in my groin"). By Ms. Boyle's account, this and other similar episodes were the factors that led to her seeking rape crisis counseling and subsequent referral to her present treating psychologist, as well as to her having left the Strong Company and initiated the above-referenced lawsuit against her former employer.

With this background and history, your firm arranged for this present psychiatric/neuropsychiatric/addiction medicine evaluation of Ms. Boyle via the circumstances and for the reasons noted above. I emphasize again that as a clinically based evaluation and report intended to address the issue of psychiatric and psychological issues, if applicable, concerning Ms. Boyle's present condition pertaining to the effects on her of her alleged sexual harassment by Mr. Strong in the latter phase of her employment with that organization, this evaluation and report are *not* intended to address the issue of whether, in fact, such harassment actually took place. Such evaluation would be legal/administrative in nature, and not within the scope of this present psychiatric/neuropsychiatric evaluation and report.

Dr. Meade reiterates the present clinical (damages) orientation and focus of the evaluation at this point, toward the end of the report.

The sources of information on which this evaluation and report are based; Ms. Boyle's background and history leading up to the period of time of the alleged workplace sexual harassment in question; my clinical observations and findings of Ms. Boyle; and my clinical diagnostic impressions are all as described above and elsewhere in records and materials available for review in this matter. That information will not be repeated in this section of this report.

> Dr. Meade refers back to Ms. Boyle's present high self-rating, in keeping with the present clinical (damages) focus of the evaluation.

With regard to my psychiatric/neuropsychiatric/addiction medicine impressions of Ms. Boyle, I note, to begin, her present rating of herself as a 9 out of 10, in terms of her overall level of functioning, satisfaction in life, productivity in life, and relationships with others. Ms. Boyle rated herself in that regard presently as doing well in life, better than she has done for most of her life leading up to the present, and in that sense, as having begun a new course of professional study and of "moving on with my life" (her words).

> The author again emphasizes that this evaluation and report do not address liability (i.e., whether or not, administratively and legally speaking, sexual harassment of Ms. Boyle actually took place) in the context of this matter.

Whether or not Ms. Boyle actually was exposed to sexual harassment by Mr. Strong in her workplace during the period of time in question, she is currently doing very well in life—better than during most of her previous life—and in that sense, is not presently experiencing consequences of her alleged workplace sexual harassment during the period of time in question, in my psychiatric/neuropsychiatric opinion. I hold this opinion with a degree of reasonable medical probability.

> Next, Dr. Meade discussed a likely bias on Ms. Boyle's part, based on her background and history. He asserts that she was primed to perceive activities as harassing, thereby affecting her perception of such activities as harassment.

In addition, given Ms. Boyle's dysfunctional and abusive background and history, to the extent that history and her experiences and feelings from that history "primed" (my word) or predisposed her to interpret activities in her workplace as sexually harassing, Ms. Boyle was very much predisposed in that way, so that her psychiatric/neuropsychiatric responses to her perceptions of sexual harassment were likely in excess of similar perceptions by an individual who had not had Ms. Boyle's life history and experiences. In that sense—again, whether or not actual sexual harassment against Ms. Boyle took place at the Strong Battery Company workplace (a factual and legal/administrative question)—her responses to her perceptions of sexual harassment in the workplace, again, were likely in excess of those experienced by an individual without her traumatic and dysfunctional background and history. Given that, from a practical clinical perspective, it would be impossible to tease out which proportion of Ms. Boyle's present psychiatric symptomatology, limited though it is, could be attributed to her perceptions of sexual harassment in the Strong Battery Company workplace.

> **Dr. Meade next reemphasizes Ms. Boyle's present high level of functioning by virtue of her not being involved in mental health treatment, in turn by virtue of his characterization of her as a survivor.**

Finally, in terms of Ms. Boyle's possible present psychiatric/neuropsychiatric symptomatology, as of this writing, Ms. Boyle is not presently involved in psychotherapy/counseling or psychiatric treatment, notwithstanding the stresses, associations, and reminders that her present litigation in the above-referenced matter is causing her. In that regard, Ms. Boyle's status as a survivor (see above) and her ability to overcome difficulties and cope with stressors is underscored, as is her own estimate of her current level of functioning (9 out of 10).

> **Last, Dr. Meade wrote the customary disclaimers, distinguishing his forensic report from a purely clinical one.**

The referenced individual was examined with reference to specific issues emanating from the original situation, in accordance with the restrictive rules concerning an independent medical examination. It is, therefore, understood that no treatment was given or suggested and that no doctor/patient relationship exists.

I aver that the information contained in this document was prepared by the undersigned and is the work of the undersigned. It is true to the best of my knowledge and information and has not been modified by anyone other than the undersigned.

Please advise me if you have questions about this present evaluation and report, or if you anticipate requiring additional services from me in connection with this matter.

Thank you very much.

Sincerely,

Steven L. Meade, MD, MS

Diplomate, American Board of Psychiatry and Neurology (P)

Certified, American Society of Addiction Medicine

Case Analysis and Outcome

Although any forensic mental health professional's consultation/evaluation is clinically based and informed, in employment law cases such as this one, that point is particularly important. The clinical mental health consultation/evaluation is not intended to address employment law or administrative questions, such as wrongful discharge, hostile work environment, or sexual harassment, but rather to assess the extent, if applicable, of the emotional and related effects of an individual's workplace experiences during the period of time in the past to his or her present clinical condition. In our experience, counsel will periodically attempt to press for a mental health expert's opinion about whether or not, for example, sexual harassment actually did occur. Such an assessment is not within the scope of a clinical evaluation, but rather is a factual question, to be addressed and determined by counsel for the parties involved. Emotional and related effects of an individual's workplace experience, on the other hand, are dangerous questions, well within the scope of a clinical evaluation.

Having made that point, a clinical aspect of Ms. Boyle's background and history has to do with her long-standing dysfunctional life, lifestyle, family, and other such aspects of her history. Notwithstanding that difficult history, and notwithstanding the question of whether or not she actually was sexually harassed in her workplace during the period of time in question, she nevertheless was doing very well clinically (in terms of her mental health and general level of functioning) at the time of her evaluation by the consulting mental health professional. In that regard, the consulting mental health professional offered the opinion that to whatever extent Ms. Boyle's workplace experiences at issue in this matter may have adversely affected her, it was not possible clinically to tease out the extent to which her present clinical condition may have been due to those experiences or to prior and subsequent stressful and difficult experiences. Ms. Boyle was doing very well clinically as of the time of the interview/examination, and damages (in the technical legal sense) were minimal, from any cause.

The evaluating psychiatrist in this case, Dr. Meade, concluded that Ms. Boyle was a survivor (his term), and that any psychiatric consequences to her workplace experiences—or to any other experiences before Dr. Meade's interview/examination of Ms. Boyle—were negligible and could not be meaningfully apportioned among one another.

This type of analysis in which the evaluator addresses damages (i.e., not liability) in these types of cases is characteristic for a role of the forensic mental health expert in civil cases. Further examples of this role will be discussed in additional cases in this section of this book.

The advocacy of the evaluating mental health professional to his expert opinion and not to either part is underscored in this case: Dr. Meade's opinions did not serve the needs of Ms. Boyle well, but he gave them as he did, and as he should. Retaining counsel chose to use Dr. Meade's report, which could not have helped his case as a report describing and emphasizing damages would have.

Although not explicit in this report, one of the pointers (Chapter 1) in attorney/expert and court/expert relationships that was central to this evaluation pertained to telephone calls and communication. In this case, retaining counsel was not prompt or efficient in communicating with Dr. Meade. This left the expert in the position of periodically having to second-guess the attorney. As an experienced expert, Dr. Meade was able to do that by anticipating the needs and time schedules (deadlines, especially) of the attorney and meeting them, thereby avoiding crises. After the case was satisfactorily resolved, the attorney was grateful to Dr. Meade for his attentiveness. Subsequent cases with Dr. Meade and the retaining attorney went more smoothly.

Ultimately, this case settled for what plaintiff's counsel characterized as "a pitiful amount of money," and defense counsel as "a ridiculously high settlement." The case did not go to trial.

Reilly v. Brower Hospital, Stanley Koch, MD, et al.

Case Overview: Professional Liability (Medical Malpractice)

This case involved a suit for medical malpractice filed by the family of a deceased, Porter Reilly, against an institution, Brower Hospital, and a doctor, Stanley Koch, MD, alleging that as a result of malpractice, the deceased, while being suicide-prone, was discharged from the hospital. He returned home and committed suicide with a samurai sword. David Turkwood, Esquire, defense counsel, retained a psychiatrist, Jeffrey R. Cameron, MD, to determine if there was any deviation from accepted standards of medical care. Dr. Cameron's report follows.

The Report

> Unlike other forensic mental health evaluations, those involving professional liability (malpractice) issues need to address both alleged liability (of the defendant) *and* damages (to the plaintiff) in these matters. That necessarily involves the review of extensive and voluminous records and materials, legal and medical, which should at least be catalogued and listed in the forensic report, if not fully synopsized. These points should be presented and discussed at the beginning of the report, since writing a report in that way may be (and in this report, is) a departure from the customary format of forensic reports as described in Chapter 1.

Following up on our telephone discussions and correspondence about the above-referenced matter, and based on the sources of information given below, I am writing you this report of my psychiatric evaluation in this matter concerning the issue of whether or not Stanley Koch, MD, deviated from accepted standards of medical care in his treatment of Porter Reilly at Brower Hospital during his psychiatric hospitalization at that facility from March 17 to March 23 in the context of Mr. Reilly's subsequent death by suicide when, after his discharge from Brower Hospital that day, "he went home and killed himself with a samurai sword" (excerpted in part from the psychiatric evaluation report of Richard Hayes, MD, to plaintiff's counsel in this matter, Terrence R. Placer, Esquire, dated October 19, XXXX).

In this evaluation—a suicide, or "wrongful death" alleged malpractice action—the plaintiff's estate brought the action, and there was nobody to interview/examine directly (in this particular case, there was also nobody with whom to do collateral interviews. Mr. Reilly, the deceased, had been an isolated individual, a loner). Therefore, the format of this particular report will not include several sections in the usual clinically based format, that is, "History," "Mental Status (Psychiatric) Examination," and "Clinical Diagnostic Impressions." Instead, the core work and analysis of this forensic evaluation consist of review of records, and a clear statement of "Summary and Opinions," based primarily on review of records. This departure from the usual format of forensic mental health reports is made clear in the introductory section—"Nature and Scope of This Evaluation"—of the report.

This present evaluation report is based on review of records, described below, and not on face-to-face interviews/examinations; the opinions expressed in it are expressed with a degree of reasonable medical probability.

Since, as a practice matter, I do not disagree to a substantial extent with points made by other physicians in other evaluations and reports in this matter (described below), and since information contained in the records and materials that I did review in connection with this evaluation and report give considerable information and details about Mr. Reilly's psychiatric and chemical dependency history leading to his outpatient treatment and emergency medical inpatient treatment at Cliff Memorial Hospital (March 13–17, XXXX) and then treatment at Brower Hospital (from March 17, XXXX), I will not reiterate details contained in those records and materials in this report.

Rather, in this report, after initially listing and discussing the records and materials that I have reviewed in connection with this evaluation and report, I will present and discuss salient points in Mr. Reilly's history leading to his treatment and subsequent suicide, and I will discuss psychiatric treatment issues relevant to the decisions made by Mr. Reilly's treatment staff (including Dr. Koch) at Brower Hospital (BH) and will conclude with my psychiatric opinion,

---

The author next discussed the legal and medical/clinical records and materials reviewed for this evaluation, as is customary with these types of reports. The writer excerpted in detail from a number of these records, in that the records were the principal sources of information for this evaluation.

held with a degree of reasonable medical probability, about "whether or not Dr. Koch met with the appropriate standards of care under the circumstances of this case" (as excerpted from your initial transmittal letter).

For further information and details contained in the records and materials that I have reviewed in connection with this evaluation and report, the reader is referred to them.

The sources of information on which this present evaluation and report are based are as follows:

1. My review of copies of legal records and materials pertaining to the above-referenced matter, as follows:

   a. "Plaintiff's Answers to Interrogatories," including Form A and Form A(1). For present purposes, Answer 7 (to Form A(1)) stated that "Generally, however, it shall be alleged that the defendant deviated from the accepted standards of care by failing to properly assess and treat decedent's suicidal condition, including discharging him while he was still an extremely high suicidal risk";

   b. A transcript of the "Deposition Upon Oral Examination" of Stanley Koch, MD, dated June XX, XXXX. To my reading, this transcript explored and discussed a variety of issues pertaining to Dr. Koch's treatment of Mr. Reilly during Mr. Reilly's hospitalization at BH during the time in question. Since an important point, in my view, concerning Dr. Koch's and the BH treatment team's treatment of Mr. Reilly during that time pertained to Mr. Reilly's suicidal intent plans, I include the following excerpt of what was known to Dr. Koch at the time of Mr. Reilly's discharge from BH:

      Q. Okay. Describe for me the difference between the Mr. Reilly who attempted to kill himself and the Mr. Reilly you discharged from the hospital.

      A. Well, I did not examine the Mr. Reilly—I'm not sure I understand the question. I did not examine Mr. Reilly before he attempted to kill himself when he was in that frame of mind, so I can't compare, so I have no reference point there, but the Mr. Reilly who was in the hospital and who was discharged seemed to feel that his suicide attempt was a mistake and he verbalized that. And he seemed to understand that his illness would take some time to be helped by the medication, and he was cooperative and willing to—you know, to let that medication take its effect without trying to kill himself again, which he considered to be a mistake.

2. My review of copies of three sets of medical records pertaining to Mr. Reilly's treatment leading up to his death by suicide on XXXX, as follows:

   a. Records from Mr. Reilly's treatment with the Blake Medical Group, his primary care providers, with various progress notes and entries from June XXXX to March XXXX. Included in these materials are notes pertaining to Mr. Reilly's medical conditions, psychiatric condition, and a discussion with Dr. Pierre Waters (psychiatrist) dated Feb. 2, XXXX, who "agrees with Lexapro 20 mg";

b. A collection of hospital records and materials concerning Mr. Reilly's psychiatric hospitalization at Cliff Memorial Hospital (CMH) from March 17, XXXX, prior to his transfer to BH on March 17, XXXX. Records and materials consist of progress notes, laboratory printouts, nursing notes, and other such records and materials and, to my reading, appear to be the complete hospital chart (hospital file, records) for this hospitalization. Mr. Reilly had been to CMH on an emergency basis after an Ambien and alcohol overdose, described in applicable records and materials as nonresponsive and comatose, treated with life support and resuscitated, and transferred to BH for psychiatric care. Mr. Reilly's diagnoses at CMH were given as "benzodiazepine overdose . . . acute respiratory failure . . . toxic effects (of) alcohol . . . suicide attempt . . . alcohol abuse . . . depression . . . gout . . . gastroesophageal reflux . . . gastroesophageal ulcer"; and

c. Another hospital chart for Mr. Reilly's treatment, this one from BH for his psychiatric hospitalization of March 17–23, XXXX (via transfer from CMH, as described above). As with the CMH records, to my reading, these materials also represent the BH chart for this hospitalization for Mr. Reilly. In the section of Dr. Koch's "Discharge Summary" for Mr. Reilly, entitled "History of Present Illness," Dr. Koch wrote that, "The patient stated that he has been increasingly depressed for the past few months. He has lost about 40 pounds. He has had trouble sleeping, difficulty concentrating, feeling like a failure, hopeless and helpless. He took an overdose of sleeping pills and some alcohol and was accidentally discovered by his wife. He also had a loaded gun in his pocket that he thought he would use if he woke up and the overdose was not successful. He left a note behind. The patient was admitted to Cliff Memorial Hospital and treated there medically before being transferred here. He stated that for about the last 10 days he has been on Lexapro from his family doctor and he has had one visit with an outpatient psychiatrist, Dr. Waters, who continued the Lexapro." In the "Nursing Assessment" section of this report, confirming the above, a "Summary Statement" indicated that "stressors include family and work. Patient is losing his business and has been lying around on the couch. Patient is becoming more depressed in the last 4–5 months. He feels like a failure and has lost 40 lbs. Patient's wife is very supportive."

Recognizing the importance of Mr. Reilly's suicidality during this hospitalization, nursing progress notes beginning on March 9, XXXX, discussed "Potential for Self-Directed Violence." On that date, a note indicates, "Patient's affect brighter and more spontaneous. Mood appears depressed. Patient socializing with peers. Patient verbalizing re: 'I was so stupid about what I did and wanted to do to myself.' Patient denies suicidal ideation. Participating well in groups. Visible on unit . . . ."

The next day, March 10, XXXX, another nursing note with the heading "Potential for Self-Directed Violence" indicated that Mr. Reilly was "calm, pleasant, social, denies SI (suicidal ideation). Feels remorseful . . . Patient has no C/O (complaints) at this time . . . " Another "Potential for Self-Directed Violence" note that same day indicated that, "Patient presents with pleasant encouraged (bright) mood, affect flat but pleasant and somewhat cheerful. Patient cooperative and present on unit. Patient visited with daughter (in college). She drove up to visit with him. Patient reported feeling embarrassed and ashamed of being on ACIS. However, patient acknowledged that daughter and wife were supportive. Patient realizes that he needs to find other ways to cope with life stressors, 'with help from clinician.' Patient acknowledged that he was an 'alcoholic.' Patient reported associating food with drinking (alcohol) and saw a difference in his appetite since arriving on the unit. Patient reports feeling much better since arriving. . . . Discussed identifying healthy coping mechanisms and continued compliance with meds. Provided education thinking about alcoholism and effects. Supportive contact offered."

The next such entry discussing "Potential for Self-Directed Violence" described Mr. Reilly as "pleasant, calm, quiet, and cooperative . . . brighter affect . . . concerns about his business . . . more focus . . . excited about going home." This note was dated March 18, XXXX. The next note concerning "Potential for Self-Directed Violence" was dated March 19, XXX, and noted that, "Patient expressed appreciation for treatment and motivation for continued care. . . . Spoke with patient's wife at 11:50 A.M. on March 19, XXXX. Patient's wife stated all hunting firearms were removed from the home on March 14 by a friend of the patient and are inaccessible." A later "Potential for Self-Directed Violence" note that day indicated that "Patient presents with brighter mood and blunted affect. Patient attends all grps (groups). Patient is visible at unit. Patient reports feeling ready for D/C (discharge) soon. Denies SI. . . . Patient calm, pleasant, and cooperative." A third "Potential for Self-Directed Violence" note that day described Mr. Reilly as "visible and somewhat social. Goes to group and on outside walks. Denies present suicidal ideation and feels he is ready for discharge which has been ordered for tomorrow."

On the date of discharge (March 23, XXXX), the "Clinician Discharge Note" indicated that "Patient presents calm, aware, oriented, and appreciative of treatment. Patient denied any potential harm to self . . . and is in agreement with the discharge plan. Motivated for aftercare."

Returning to Dr. Koch's "Discharge Summary" for Mr. Reilly, several parts of this summary described and discussed Mr. Reilly's mental state, depression, and suicidality. The "Mental Status Examination" section indicated that "on admission, he is an alert and oriented white male who looks to be his stated age or somewhat older. He complains of severe difficulty sleeping and initial and intermittent waking too early. No hallucinations or delusions. Minimal racing thoughts. Poor memory and concentration. Feelings of hopelessness and helplessness. He denies being particularly suicidal on admission." Mr. Reilly's "Hospital Course" section of this summary indicated that, "During the patient's hospital stay, he was continued on Lexapro 20 mg. It was explained to him the medical concept of depression as an illness. It was explained to him the negative perceptions of himself in the world as well as the physical manifestations of this disease and that the medication that he had started on was a good one for this illness, but that it would take some time, in fact, a number of weeks to really provide relief for him and to be patient about that. While in the hospital, the patient was stable and cooperative with the therapeutic process. He denied being suicidal. He stated that he felt that was a stupid thing that he did. He felt, in fact, rather ashamed of what he had done in terms of trying to harm himself. The patient engaged in self-reflection and felt that he had been rather isolative from his family and his wife previously because of other experiences that he had in the past and that he felt closer to his wife and family and wanted to work on that relationship. Patient was an outdoorsman, hunting and fishing. He apparently has some firearms in the home that he used for hunting. I contacted his wife, and between his wife and the patient, they got a friend to come over and take the firearms out of the house. The local police had the original firearm apparently that had been in his pocket. The patient's mood remained depressed during his hospital stay but, again, not suicidal. He seemed to understand the way the medications would gradually be working. He seemed to be able to benefit from the support of others in his environment, including his family, the patients, and his colleagues and friends at work. The patient was more open about his history of drinking. He attended some alcohol abuse oriented meetings during his hospital stay and began to see himself as someone who had a drinking problem and began to feel comfortable in the support of those types of groups. The patient was discharged on Lexapro and to be followed up in the outpatient MICA (Mentally Ill Chemical Abuser) Program."

Dr. Koch's "Discharge Diagnoses" for Mr. Reilly at that time were: "Axis I (of the *DSM-IV-TR,* described in further detail below): Major depression. Axis II: None. Axis III: Gout. Gastroesophageal reflux disease status post diverticulitis surgery. Hepatitis C infection. Axis IV: Four. Axis V Global Assessment of Functioning: 20/10. . ." (the handwritten list of discharge diagnoses also included "S/P (status post) Overdose";

3. My review of copies of psychiatric evaluation reports in this matter for plaintiff's counsel, as follows:

   a. A report by Charles B. West, MD, retained as plaintiff's expert forensic evaluator, dated XXXX, and sent to plaintiff's counsel. Dr. West's opinion in this matter was that "these deviations from the good and proper standards of medical and psychiatric treatment were the cause of the death of Mr. Porter Reilly by suicide on the same day he was released from Brower Hospital on March 23, XXXX." Dr. West identified "four specific deviations" from acceptable medical and psychiatric practice by the treatment and care rendered at Brower Hospital from March 17 to March 23, XXXX:

      1. Brower Hospital staff and physicians failed to recognize the high suicidal risks of Porter Reilly in discharging him from the hospital on March 23.

2. Mr. Porter Reilly was discharged from the hospital without his underlying psychiatric condition, major depressive disorder, being properly treated. There was a failure to recognize the serious suicidal potential and ensure the safety of Mr. Porter Reilly by maintaining him in the hospital until his depression could be brought under sufficient treatment to ensure his safety.

3. Brower Hospital staff and physicians did not do a comprehensive medical workup in relation to Mr. Reilly having hepatitis C and consider the effects this would have in relation to his depression, nor take into consideration the interaction in relation to the medications used for treatment of his psychiatric disturbance.

4. Brower Hospital staff and physicians failed to conduct sequential suicide risk assessments over the course of time and to recognize the high potential risk for suicide in Mr. Porter Reilly and therefore keep him in the hospital until his condition had been brought under sufficient control to ensure his safety.

Attached to this report were several pages of receipts and lists of expenses pertaining to Mr. Reilly. For further information and details, the reader is referred to materials and report;

b. A supplemental report by Dr. West to plaintiff's counsel, this one dated October XXXX, and based on Dr. West's review of Dr. Koch's deposition (above). After initially listing several areas of what may be characterized as deviations and deficiencies by Dr. Koch in his treatment of Mr. Reilly, Dr. West offered the "Opinion" that "there were significant departures from good and acceptable psychiatric/medical practice in the care and treatment rendered by Dr. Koch of Mr. Porter Reilly when he was a patient under his psychiatric treatment at Brower Hospital from March 17 to March 23, XXXX." Dr. West next listed and discussed these areas of deviation, to my reading, focusing on risk factors and statistical/epidemiologic factors, to my reading. Dr. West wrote, for example, that "Dr. Koch did not have any contact with Mrs. Reilly during the hospitalization. Mrs. Reilly was never included in any discussions regarding the types of weapons Mr. Reilly had in his possession. The risk of suicide increases 40% in an individual who owns a gun. In this case, although the guns were addressed, a simple discussion with Mrs. Reilly would have indicated the presence of a samurai sword, which ultimately is as lethal as a gun. In addition, Mrs. Reilly was not apprised of her husband's condition or given any guidance particularly what to look for in the first 48 hours, which is a time period of greater risk for suicide." Dr. West also wrote that, "Dr. Koch offered the opinion that Mr. Reilly was 'not particularly suicidal.' This, in the face of what is obvious clinical evidence to the contrary, underscores that Dr. Koch did not conduct adequate suicide risk assessments. Dr. Koch offered the opinion that Mr. Reilly was psychologically better on discharge. However, the records do not give evidence that this is the case." Dr. West concluded the supplemental report by writing. "In review of the records, it is my opinion within reasonable medical certainty that Dr. Koch did not exercise a degree of care consistent with that of a trained psychiatrist respectably employing prudence and meeting standards of care. It is my considered opinion that this was a deviation of negligence and he did not exercise a standard of care that would be similarly employed by other psychiatrists under similar clinical circumstance. In my opinion, these deviations from good and proper standards of medical and psychiatric treatment were the direct proximate cause of the unfortunate death by suicide of Mr. Porter Reilly on the day he was discharged from Brower Hospital on March 23, XXXX";

c. Another psychiatric report by Dr. Richard Hayes to plaintiff's counsel concerning the question of "whether the care rendered to Mr. Porter Reilly by Brower Hospital fell below acceptable standards of care, and whether there is any causal relationship between the care rendered by Brower Hospital and Mr. Reilly's death by suicide on March 23, XXXX" (excerpted from the introductory paragraph of this report). This report was dated November 11, XXXX. After initially listing the records and materials that Dr. West had reviewed in his evaluation and giving a "Summary of Relevant Records" (including Mr. Reilly's CMH and BH hospitalizations), Dr. Hayes gave a "Medical-Clinical Formulation, reasoning and opinion." Dr. Hayes here focused on Mr. Reilly's risk factors, in retrospect, for suicide, as did Dr. West, and he also gave the opinion that "he (Mr. Reilly) was admitted to Brower Hospital two days later, and six days after that, he was discharged and successfully killed himself on March 23, XXXX. His time period on Lexapro was simply inadequate to determine if the medication was going to work and to what degree. The time period on Lexapro frequently requires 8–12 weeks of treatment at an adequate dose for a response, meaning a 50% reduction in symptoms. Mr. Reilly clearly had not reached even this level of therapeutic success at the time of this discharge." Dr. Hayes also offered the opinion that "the staff and physicians at Brower Hospital did not appropriately evaluate, appreciate, or treat the risk factors for suicide presented by Mr. Reilly. These include the following:

1. The diagnosis of major depression carries with it a significant danger of suicidality, especially when not adequately treated, and Mr. Reilly was not adequately treated psychopharmacologically with Lexapro, as previously noted.

2. Mr. Reilly was in a category of patients that carry a high suicide risk. Males are known to complete the act of suicide more successfully and at a greater rate than females. Suicidality increases with age and with a history of recent loss. Mr. Reilly felt that he was losing his business and his financial livelihood and everything associated with that.

3. Mr. Reilly also had a serious, planned, premeditated suicide attempt, which was not impulsive in nature. He wrote a note, planned an overdose of pills, and was accidentally found by his wife. He had a backup plan in that he had a loaded gun, which he planned to use if the pills were not successful in killing him. The gun certainly would provide a lethal means for suicide.

4. The role of alcohol in this patient's life was never clearly defined
    by the hospital, though it was strongly suspected that alcohol was
    more of a problem for Mr. Reilly than he was admitting. The addi-
    tion of alcohol problems increases the danger of suicidality.
5. Of particular significance is that Mr. Reilly masked his suicidal-
    ity on a previous occasion to Dr. Waters, to whom he denied ac-
    tive or passive suicidal ideation or intent. Three days after seeing
    Dr. Waters, he made a very serious and planned suicide attempt.
    With this history of having fooled Dr. Waters, Brower Hospital, its
    staff, and its physicians should have had a high degree of suspi-
    cion that Mr. Reilly would feign good mental health with them as
    well, deny suicidality, and upon discharge would make another
    suicide attempt. This is exactly what he did. The hospital, its staff
    and physicians, therefore, did not use this known past history to
    prevent this deadly occurrence. Instead, Mr. Reilly was prema-
    turely discharged from the hospital before it could be determined
    if his antidepressant medication would work, or to what degree it
    would work."

Dr. Hayes concluded his report by offering his "medical opinion, with
reasonable medical certainty, that Brower Hospital, its staff, and its physicians, in the treatment of Mr. Reilly, did not exercise the reasonable
judgment and standard of care expected of the practice of clinical psychiatry in the community. It is also my medical opinion, with reasonable
medical certainty, that there is a direct proximate causal relationship
between the clinical treatment provided by Brower Hospital, its physician and staff, and the subsequent death by suicide of Mr. Reilly";

d. A copy of another report to Mr. Placer, plaintiff's counsel, this one au-
    thored by Michael Ryan, MD, and dated March 8, XXXX; this report was
    accompanied by a copy of Dr. Ryan's resume.
    After initially indicating that he had been "asked to review the medi-
    cal records of Mr. Porter Reilly from the perspective of whether there
    was negligence on the part of Dr. Koch and whether deviations in the
    standard of care directly caused the suicidal death of Mr. Reilly," Dr.
    Ryan listed the records and documents that he had reviewed, gave
    an autobiographical sketch and fee schedule for himself, and a "Brief
    Summary of Case." He next reviewed the CMH and BH records, fo-
    cusing on areas of particular concern to him, leading to his opinions.
    Dr. Ryan identified several "Major Concerns Re: Negligence," including
    "alcohol use, handgun charges, lethal methods of self-harm at home,
    and psychiatric care provided by Dr. Koch." Dr. Ryan noted several
    medical and psychiatric points, for example, including Mr. Reilly's hep-
    atitis C and his 40-pound weight loss leading to his initial overdose
    and hospitalization, Dr. Koch's not having spoken with Dr. Waters (who
    first treated Mr. Reilly for depression via referral from Mr. Reilly's pri-
    mary care physician, Dr. Stone), Dr. Koch's not having read Mr. Reilly's
    suicide note, and others. Dr. Ryan did describe a total of eight "devia-
    tions from the standard of care by Dr. Koch," in his opinion, giving the

"Clinical and Scientific Basis for My Opinions" in subsequent pages of his report, citing a number referenced from the professional literature. He also indicated later in the report that "I have grave concerns about the negligent assessment, treatment and management provided by Dr. Koch, as illustrated below," describing them in several areas, including "Psychosocial and Environmental Problems," "Global Assessment of Functioning," "Risk Assessment," Discharge Planning," and "Associated Depressive Symptoms." He gave a list of what he characterized as 10 specific areas of deviations "from the standards of care in the assessment, treatment, management, and discharge planning in one or more of the following areas."

Dr. Ryan concluded in his report and opinions, as follows: "Despite indicating in his deposition that he was aware of the majority of Mr. Reilly's risk factors associated with increased risk for suicide, Dr. Koch failed to integrate them into his assessment of Mr. Reilly and the importance of coordinating his discharge and discharge plans with his primary care physician (Dr. Stone) and with Mr. Reilly's wife and his family. Dr. Koch's failure to assess the possibility of suicide led to a failure to foresee the potential risk of suicide, which resulted in a failure to investigate and ensure appropriate safeguards in the outpatient setting. These failures were the direct proximate cause of Mr. Reilly's suicidal death within two hours of being discharged from Brower Hospital on March 23, XXXX. Based upon the information provided to me, it is my opinion that Dr. Koch was negligent in his treatment of Mr. Reilly. Dr. Koch's failure to obtain an adequate history and to foresee the ongoing risk for suicide by Mr. Reilly represents deviations from the acceptable standard of care. It is my further opinion that if Dr. Koch had read the medical records, obtained clinical information from the other physicians involved in Mr. Reilly's recent care, spoken with family members, appropriately educated the family members about Mr. Reilly's ongoing risk for suicide; and had taken appropriate precautions to limit Mr. Reilly's access to lethal means, foreseen the possibility of ongoing risk for suicide, and made appropriate postdischarge plans, that with a reasonable degree of medical and psychiatric certainty, the suicide of Mr. Reilly on March 23, XXXX would have been prevented"; and

4. My knowledge, background, training, and experience in psychiatry, neuropsychiatry, addiction medicine, and forensic psychiatry.

Going directly to the "Summary and Opinions" section of this report from the record review completes the departure from the usual clinically based forensic report format endorsed in this book (Chapter 1). That point should be made early in the report, as an introduction to the report, and reiterated at the end, as it is in this report.

Summary and Opinions

Without reiterating the extensive background, history, and details discussed above and elsewhere in records and materials available for review in this matter, and acknowledging again that I do not substantially disagree with the information, data, and points made by Dr. West (in his two reports), Dr. Hayes, and Dr. Ryan in their reports, I note, as also mentioned above, that to a large extent, all of these individuals used the concept of risk factors, in retrospect, in arriving at their opinions concerning Dr. Koch and BH having deviated from accepted standards of medical and psychiatric care, and in inferring a causal relationship between that deviation and Mr. Reilly's subsequent death. Their analyses are, in my view, retrospective to some extent, in that such facts as Mr. Reilly's having had a samurai sword at his home (despite indications that his potential suicide weapons had been removed in anticipation of his returning home) could not have been known prior to his discharge from BH. Such demographic risk factors as Mr. Reilly's age, his business reversals, his alcohol problem (which was known to Dr. Koch by virtue of aftercare arrangements with an MICA program), his diagnosis of depression, his prior suicide attempt and medical treatment at CMH, and numerous other facts and factors were known to Dr. Koch and BH staff during Mr. Reilly's course of treatment at CMH. As a practical matter, whether or not a given demographic factor will predict any given outcome in any individual (e.g., whether depression, lethality, age, gender, and so forth will predict completed suicide) is not methodologically, to my understanding, something that can be predicted with certainty for any individual. Therefore, to the extent that demographic and risk factors for completed suicide form the basis of the opinions of Dr. West, and Dr. Hayes, I respectfully disagree that they can be applied with certainty to a specific individual (such as Mr. Reilly).

After giving his first reason for disputing the opinion of the plaintiff's expert psychiatrist, Dr. Cameron then presented and discussed other bases for his disagreement with Dr. West's opinions.

From a clinical perspective, a number of indications exist in the record that Mr. Reilly had regarded the overdose suicide attempt that had led to his hospitalization at CMH as a mistake, in retrospect, and as something that he regretted (as described, for example, in the excerpts from BH records described above). To my reading of applicable records and materials, Mr. Reilly was consistent in his discussions with BH staff that he was no longer suicidal during his hospitalization at BH, and that he was looking forward to returning home and getting on with his life. In retrospect and by inference, this was not the case; however, from a practical perspective, in order to have made clinical decisions that were contrary to Mr. Reilly's actual expressions, comments, and wishes would have required that his treating staff either have been clairvoyant or have been able to "read his (Mr. Reilly's) mind" (my words) during that hospitalization, which of course is not possible. Making decisions not based on risk factors, the types of historical events that are described by Drs. West, Hayes, and Ryan, and in retrospect making clinical decisions based on those types of information and observations in an individual case would not, in my psychiatric/neuropsychiatric/

addiction medicine opinion, held with a degree of reasonable medical probability, have been advisable, since such decisions would have been contrary, again in retrospect, to Mr. Reilly's wishes and to general psychiatric treatment goals of encouraging individuals to resume their lives and to be treated psychiatrically in the least restrictive alternative available and appropriate to them (i.e., outpatient rather than inpatient, when clinically indicated and appropriate).

To have retained Mr. Reilly on a voluntary basis at BH following the time of his actual discharge (recognizing and accepting, again, that he probably had planned all along to attempt suicide on discharge from CMH, a plan that he did not reveal to anybody) would have gone against his wishes and would have maintained his dependent relationship on hospitalization, a situation that is generally not advocated by clinicians except in the case of the chronically institutionalized mentally ill who cannot cope with life outside such institutions. To have involuntarily hospitalized Mr. Reilly at that time (and transferred him to a facility that can accommodate such involuntarily hospitalized individuals) would have been disruptive to Mr. Reilly's treatment at the time and would have also continued his dependency on an institutional setting. In any event, such decisions at that time, in retrospect, would have had to have been made on the basis of risk factors and historical events, and on the basis of Mr. Reilly's apparent clinical status at BH and on his wishes.

In summary, and recognizing that in retrospect, the historical points and risk factors described by Drs. West, Hayes, and Ryan were accurate and applicable to Mr. Reilly's situation at the time, his intended lethality was only known, in retrospect, to himself. To have made clinical decisions not to have discharged him to an MICA aftercare program at the time would have assumed that Dr. Koch and the BH staff, again, could have been somehow clairvoyant about Mr. Reilly's behaviors of two hours after his actual discharge, or that they could have been able to "read his mind" (again, my words) with regard to his wishes and stated intent (his stated intent having been not to commit suicide).

Finally, Dr. Cameron reiterated his expert opinion in this matter briefly and succinctly, bringing his report full circle.

For these reasons, I respectfully disagree with the opinions of Dr. West, Dr. Hayes, and Dr. Ryan with regard to Dr. Koch and BH having deviated from accepted standards of medical and psychiatric care of Mr. Reilly during the period of time in question, and that these purported deviations were the proximate cause of his death by suicide.

Dr. Cameron wrote the customary disclaimer, distinguishing his forensic report from a purely clinical one.

I aver that the information contained in this document was prepared by the undersigned and is the work of the undersigned. It is true to the best of my knowledge and information and has not been modified by anyone other than the undersigned.

Please advise me if you have questions about this present evaluation and report, or if you anticipate requiring additional services from me in connection with this matter.

Thank you very much.

Sincerely,

Jeffrey R. Cameron, MD

Diplomate, American Board of Psychiatry and Neurology (P)

Certified, American Society of Addiction Medicine

Case Analysis and Outcome

Unlike the usual role of the forensic mental health expert in consultations/evaluations in civil matters, the role of the consulting/evaluating mental health expert in professional liability (malpractice) matters such as this one is to determine both liability and damages. For that reason, as a practical matter, when plaintiff's counsel seeks to obtain expert consultation in such matters, counsel usually seeks an expert in the same field or discipline, or in a field or discipline as close as possible to that of the defendant clinician, for the consultation/evaluation.

In this particular case—a psychiatric medical malpractice case—one of the consulting experts, Dr. Cameron (a consultant/evaluator for defense counsel in this case) was a psychiatrist, the same discipline as that of Dr. Koch, the defendant. Dr. Cameron's opinion was a "second opinion" (the authors' characterization) to that of Dr. West and Dr. Ryan, forensic mental health experts for the deceased plaintiff. In addressing the issue of both liability and damages, Dr. Cameron offered the opinion, in effect, that since there was no liability on the part of the defendant physician and hospital, there could have been and were no damages resulting from the activities of the defendant physician and hospital.

Forensic mental health experts often conceptualize the elements of professional liability in four "Ds," as follows:

1. The clinician had a *Duty* to treat the patient, or client;
2. The clinician was *Deviant* in his/her treatment of that patient/client;
3. *Damages* resulted from that allegedly deviant treatment; and
4. The damages were a *Direct*, or "proximate" (in legal parlance) result of the damages to the patient/client under treatment.

In an unusual turn of events, this case went to trial. It did not settle because of what defense *and* plaintiff's counsel both characterized as "bullheaded intransigence" on their clients' and their own parts. A jury trial found for the defense, offering that there was an insufficient causal link between Dr. Koch's and the hospital's treatment of Mr. Reilly and his subsequent suicide. This outcome is not unusual, in our experience: Although many medical malpractice cases do not go to trial, those that do are often decided in favor of the defense.

I/M/O Greta Palmer, An Alleged Incompetent

Case Overview: Civil Commitment—Mental Health Law

The questions in this case were, first, the determination of competence/incompetence of an elderly woman, Greta Palmer, and, second, the possibility of civil commitment of that individual. Counsel for the family members requesting such determinations, Donald Webster, Esquire, retained the psychiatrist, Regina Harrison, MD, PhD, who prepared the following report.

The Report

Returning to the conventional core format of forensic mental health reports, this one addresses two bread-and-butter topics in civil forensic evaluations: (a) general competency in an elderly person; and (b) civil commitment of that person. These two issues are clearly presented at the beginning of this report, as are the salient features of records and materials reviewed for the evaluation and the other sources of information on which the evaluation is based.

Following up on our telephone discussions and correspondence about the above-referenced matter, and based on the sources of information given below, I am writing you this report of my psychiatric/neuropsychiatric/addiction medicine evaluation of Ms. Greta Palmer in this matter.

This report is provided at your request, and is intended to give you my psychiatric/neuropsychiatric/addiction medicine opinion—held with a degree of reasonable medical probability—about whether or not inferences about Ms. Palmer's underlying mental state and psychiatric/neuropsychiatric/addiction medicine condition as of the time of my interview/examination of her (at the Forest Hills Facility, a nursing home in Bakertown, on July 5, XXXX) and for the reasonable foreseeable future after that would support a legal/court determination concerning Ms. Palmer's general mental competency, ability to take care of herself and her affairs independently (including such activities of daily living [ADLs], in turn including handling her finances, cooking and cleaning, purchasing such necessities as clothing and food), about whether or not she exhibits the type of cognitive capacity and insight and judgment necessary to conduct herself and her affairs on a day-to-day basis, conduct herself and her affairs in a safe and secure way (e.g., not leave the stove on for long periods of time, and generating a fire hazard as a result), and so forth. All of these points are intended to address the forensic psychiatric/neuropsychiatric/addiction medicine issue of whether or not Ms. Palmer may be considered generally competent, according to applicable state law, as I understand that law.

In addition to my own face-to-face interview/examination of Ms. Palmer at Forest Hills, this interview/examination was also conducted with Reginald B. Watkins, MD (a licensed physician, with training and certification in Occupational Medicine, with whom I have done a number of such competency evaluations over the years), and with Ms. Palmer's daughter, Ms. Grace Burns, who was present throughout most of the interview/examination, at Ms. Palmer's request. Dr. Watkins will be issuing his own independent evaluation report in this matter.

> Clinical records and materials are particularly relevant in this type of case, both in terms of distant history and of more recent history leading up to the present. The latter is especially important concerning the evaluee's recent and present level of functioning (as recorded on the "GAF Scale Score" of the *DSM-IV-TR*), and concerning probability—if so—of future dangerousness (for civil commitment purposes). The salient features of this clinical history should be summarized and clearly presented.

This report will also address the issue of whether or not from a clinical perspective, Ms. Palmer warrants involuntary hospitalization (civil commitment) for reasons to be discussed in further detail below.

With the above introduction to the nature and scope of this present evaluation and report, the sources of information on which this evaluation and report are based are as follows:

1. My review of copies of medical/psychiatric/clinical records and materials provided to me by your office in connection with this matter, as follows:

   a. Consultation, progress, and related notes from Ms. Palmer's hospitalization at the West Haven Hospital (WHH), where Ms. Palmer had been psychiatrically hospitalized under emergency circumstances in May XXXX, prior to her transfer to Forest Hills the following month, for continued treatment.

      Without reiterating details contained in these notes, they describe her having been admitted under urgent circumstances on May 8, XXXX, in a debilitated and intoxicated condition, complicated by her history of cognitive impairment. Ms. Palmer's psychiatric history of previous treatment at hospitalizations as well as her treatment for spinal problems, diabetes mellitus, gastritis (alcoholic), and other such chronic medical problems are described in these notes.

      For further information and details contained in these records and materials, the reader is referred to them;

   b. What appears to be an Admission Note for Ms. Palmer to the WHH, stating the following:

      "Agitated, screaming out loudly. Patient is a 92 y.o. married female who was brought in by ambulance after Pt.'s [patient's] daughter called 911. Pt. reported to her daughter that she 'didn't' feel well, namely feeling weak for the past two days, not sleeping adequately. Patient denied reduced PO [oral] intake, however mentioned that, 'I am in depression. When I am depressed, I would take a shot of vodka and orange juice at bedtime.' Patient denied suicidal ideations at present time; however, there is a history when she attempted suicide a few years ago by O.D.-meds (doesn't remember which ones). Currently, she complained about having a lot of troubles . . . husband fell down and sustained a fracture of the spine. Pt. husband currently at Newburn Hospital for rehab for a few weeks. Patient's aide quitted taking care of her 2–3 days. She was left alone during these days and probably decompensated and c/o [complained of] weakness to her daughter . . . Past Psychiatric History . . . followed by Kramer Psychiatric Clinic at Greymoore Hospital (GH). Last time saw a psychiatrist two weeks ago. Prozac 10 mg QD [daily] and Lorazepam 1 mg BID.

Hx [history] of 1 prior suicide attempt (few years ago by OD). Past Medical History: Parkinson's Disease. History of ETOH [alcohol] abuse (1 detox at Milton General Hospital). Social History: Family members: Doctors (including psychiatrists). Mental Status Examination: Alert, calm, cooperative, oriented times three. Speech calm, normal rate and rhythm. Mood—depressed. Affect—restricted. 0/3 recall, reduced cognitive abilities (did poorly with sevens) not psychotic currently. Not suicidal . . . Axis I: Depressive Disorder NOS [Not otherwise Specified]. Cognitive Disorder, NOS. R/O [Rule Out] Benzodiazepine dependence."

c. For present purposes, a "To Whom It May Concern" letter about Ms. Palmer's issues pertaining to her cognitive capacity was written by Thomas Shah, MD (Ms. Palmer's attending psychiatrist during her hospitalization at WHH), which stated the following:

This letter is to inform you that the above-named 90-year-old female patient was admitted to West Haven Hospital on May 8, XXXX. The patient was evaluated by Psychiatry on June 12, XXXX, to address the issues of capacity for decision making for discharge planning and living independently. Based on our evaluation and collateral information obtained, we found this patient to have cognitive impairment that would interfere with her ability to live alone and care for herself. Having no ability to participate in discharge planning or live independently, the patient needs to be discharged to a supervised setting with decision making to be addressed by her healthcare proxy and/or next of kin" (for practical purposes, to my understanding, this is her daughter, Ms. Grace Burns, who currently has power of attorney over her mother);

d. A collection of 19 nursing assessment documents for Ms. Palmer, completed by Brenda Reid, RN, of the Forest Hills facility, dated October 15, XXXX.

To my understanding, this assessment was completed prior to Ms. Palmer's transfer from WHH to Forest Hills. For present purposes, specific comments concerning Ms. Palmer's cognitive capacity were

made in the "AM/PM Prep" document ("Assistance into bed at night
. . . frequent checks throughout the day . . . overnight checks"); under
"Mentation" ("Regular Orientation and her intervention/supervision
outside facility in [illegible] minimal to moderate impairment"); "Behavioral Management" ("Minimal Intervention/Occasional Monitoring
. . . May wander, occasional episode, minimal monitoring"); "Medica-
tions/Service" ("Medication assistance with 10+ total medications . . .
Significant management in ordering, changing medications with/from
professionals [more than two hours per month] . . . Does not utilize
Unit-Dose method, must complete full set-up of medications"); and
"Comments" ("POA 24/7 to assist with adjusting with facility. POA to
provide assistance to ADLs. 11/24/06 Continues to have POA to assist
with all ADLs w/K to do medication");

e. A collection of nine sets of Progress Notes by Keith Marion (Ms. Palm-
    er's treating Psychiatrist at Forest Hills), dated August 1, XXXX (the
    intake note); August 8, XXXX; August 14, XXXX; August 28, XXXX; Sep-
    tember 5, XXXX; September 27, XXXX; December 5, XXXX; December
    12, XXXX; and December 18, XXXX. Included in these materials were
    several health insurance claim forms for these sessions.

    In these notes, to my reading, Dr. Marion described Ms. Palmer's
    background and history (including psychiatric disorder of major de-
    pressive disorder, with dementia NOS and R/O alcohol abuse). In his
    progress notes, Dr. Marion described Ms. Palmer's several psychotropic
    medications (including antipsychotics and antidepressants), her con-
    flicted marriage, her suicidal feelings ("so I'll die, slit my throat and get
    it over with," recorded on August 14, XXXX), her desire to return to her
    home, her depression and anxiety, her confusion and alcohol use, and
    other such aspects of her background and history as also described in
    the WHH notes;

f. Several outpatient laboratory and ECG notes for Ms. Palmer for Sep-
    tember, XXXX, presumably taken as part of her treatment and care at
    Forest Hills; and

g. Another collection of records and materials concerning Ms. Palmer's
    care at Forest Hills, consisting of copies of Physician's Order Sheets
    and Medex (dispensing) records for August through September, XXXX.
    The "Diagnosis" given on the "Partners Physician's Orders Sheet" of
    November 16, XXXX, includes Alzheimer's Disease, hypertension, and
    gastroesophageal reflux disease (GERD). At that time, Ms. Palmer's
    ordered medications were Folate, Prozac, Lopressor, Ecotrin, Multi-
    Vitamins, Nexium, Ativan, Norvasc, and Risperdal; Alprazolam (Xanax)
    was discontinued at that time. These medications, to my reading, have
    been continued through December XXXX, with the exception of Pro-
    zac (discontinued) and with the addition of Lexapro (another SSRI
    antidepressant agent).

    For further information and details contained in all of these records
    and materials, the reader is referred to them;

2. My psychiatric/neuropsychiatric/addiction medicine interview/examination
    of Ms. Palmer, which was conducted for the most part with her daughter, Ms.
    Grace Burns, and Dr. Watkins in attendance;

3. Owing to Ms. Palmer's cognitive limitations, I administered only one of a battery of standardized psychological, chemical dependency, and related tests and inventories. This one was the Mini-Mental State Examination or MMSE, with which she had considerable difficulty, and which she did not want to complete. Her performance on that test will be discussed in further detail below; and

> **Dr. Harrison's particular area of expertise is geriatric psychiatry, a point made at this early point in her report.**

4. My knowledge, background, training, and experience in psychiatry and neuropsychiatry, addiction medicine, psychiatry—and for present purposes, in particular—my work and experience over the years with individuals with various types of dementia and brain damage, congenital and acquired, as in Ms. Palmer's situation, to be discussed in further detail below.

> Augmenting information contained in Ms. Palmer's clinical records, this particular history points out her long-standing history of dysfunctional psychosocial problems, alcoholism, and more recently dementia, aggravated by her continuing alcohol use. This culminated in Ms. Palmer's institutionalization, and set a foundation for the evaluator's "Summary and Opinions" about the two forensic mental health issues addressed in this evaluation.

History

Ms. Greta Palmer is a 92-year-old (DOB: December 18, XXXX) widowed and remarried white female, most recently (prior to her hospitalization at WHH and her subsequent transfer to Forest Hills) living with her second husband (Charles Palmer, CPA, 80 years old) in a large private home that Ms. Palmer owns. As described by Ms. Palmer's daughter (from whom a good deal of the historical information about Ms. Palmer came, because of Ms. Palmer's cognitive impairment and memory loss, and consequent difficulty in communicating), Ms. Palmer and her husband are currently estranged (by virtue of her placement at Forest Hills) and in the process of divorcing; as of this writing, it is my understanding that her husband is contemplating leaving the family home or has already done so.

Ms. Palmer herself is one in a sibship of three: Her older brother, Wayne Palmer, died at the age of 85, and was possibly diagnosed with bipolar disorder during his life; her sister, Betty White, died at the age of 70. Both Ms. Palmer's brother and sister were married, and have adult children. Ms. Palmer herself had been married to Mr. Alan Bickler, who died of a stroke and a heart attack at 56 years of age; she has one daughter by that relationship, Grace Bickler

Burns, age 60, married to Vincent Burns, MD. Ms. Burns and her husband have a 27-year-old son and a 25-year-old daughter, the latter of whom is described by her mother (Mrs. Grace Burns) as having emotional problems, and as being "bipolar."

According to her daughter, Ms. Palmer was born and raised in Plaindale, graduated at a young age from Lincoln Hall High School, and attended and graduated from Tisdale University. She worked outside the home for a number of years, married her first husband, and had her children. That husband, Mr. Alan Bickler, died, and in XXXX she remarried to Mr. Charles Palmer. Mr. Palmer had also been previously married, and has three adult children.

> **At this point in the report, Dr. Harrison began to discuss factors in Ms. Palmer's history pertaining to her subsequent cognitive impairment. These factors were of particular importance in evaluating Ms. Palmer's mental competence.**

According to Ms. Burns, her mother's relationship with Mr. Palmer was marked during its later years by his having to accommodate her ongoing and severe alcoholism, in what Ms. Burns described as an increasingly dysfunctional relationship. During one period of their marriage, reportedly, Mr. Palmer was convicted of financial charges, and was incarcerated in a federal prison for a number of years.

In more recent years, as Ms. Palmer's dementia and disability and alcoholism worsened, and it was necessary for Mr. Palmer to take care of her in his aging years, the relationship deteriorated further.

According to Ms. Burns, this situation culminated in July of XXXX, when Mr. Palmer tripped and sustained a back injury, making it more difficult for him to take care of his wife. With that history, he reportedly filed for divorce from her on September 9, XXXX, after Ms. Palmer had been transferred from WHH to Forest Hills (she was reluctant to do this, and agreed to her present placement at her daughter's urging; according to Ms. Burns, her mother has consistently resisted that placement).

> **Dr. Harrison concluded the "History" section of her report with a brief discussion of Ms. Palmer's present circumstances and clinical condition.**

Presently, and for about the past four months, Ms. Palmer has lived at Forest Hills; has had frequent contact with her daughter, Ms. Burns; and has had inconsistent help from *per diem* attendants (according to Ms. Burns, her mother has generally been offensive with such individuals, and they have quit). She is on multiple psychotropic and nonpsychotropic medications for her several medical conditions (described above) and has consistently described wanting to return to live independently at her home and not remain at Forest Hills.

For further information and details about Ms. Palmer's background and history, leading up to her present placement at Forest Hills, the reader is referred to applicable records and materials, as described above.

Since the crux of this evaluation is on Ms. Palmer's present and future (for the reasonably foreseeable future, both in terms of her ability to take care of herself—her general competency—and her dangerousness or potential for dangerousness) mental states, the "Mental Status (Psychiatric) Examination" section of the report is particularly important for this type of forensic evaluation. A vivid account, with behavioral examples and quotations from the evaluee, is given in this report. These observations, in turn, support the evaluator's "Clinical Diagnostic Impressions" of Ms. Palmer, and lead to the evaluator's "Summary and Opinions."

Mental Status (Psychiatric) Examination

As indicated above, most of the interview/examination of Ms. Palmer was conducted at Forest Hills with Dr. Watkins, and also with Ms. Burns present. The reason for Ms. Burns's presence was that she told me that her mother would not agree to be interviewed/examined if she were not present. A good deal of the history was obtained from Ms. Burns rather than Ms. Palmer, owing to Ms. Palmer's cognitive limitations, memory impairments, and other communicative inabilities to relate her history and present situation to us.

I introduced myself to her, ascertained her understanding of the purpose and scope of the interview/examination, and advised her of the likelihood nonconfidential nature of the evaluation. She told me this was acceptable to her. We then proceeded with the interview/examination.

Ms. Palmer presented as a thin, slight, well-developed, well-nourished white female with reddish hair, black slacks, a purple sweater, and slippers. She seemed quite frail, and had difficulty walking: Her gait was shuffling, a Parkinsonian gait. Ms. Palmer's hands were arthritic, and throughout the interview/examination, she seemed confused about most topics that we discussed (including her family relationships with her deceased husband and her present husband, her children and grandchildren, her deceased brother and sister and their children, her location, her present relationship with her husband and her understanding about whether or not he was going to be moving out of the home, and other such topics as discussed in further detail below).

Ms. Palmer's affect was blunted throughout the interview/examination, although on several occasions (for example, when I administered the MMSE to her), she seemed irritable and angry, and not cooperative with my administering that test. (Dr. Watkins, on the other hand, did not administer such tests to Ms. Palmer, and throughout the interview/examination, she was pleasant and cooperative with him.)

Allowing for Ms. Palmer's difficulty in communicating, there did not appear to be any indication of thought disorder or psychotic processes or symptomatology (such as hallucinations, delusions, loosening of associations, and so forth) during this interview/examination. *The most striking parts of Ms.*

Palmer's mental status examination were her cognitive impairments and limitations [emphasis added], described next.

Cognitively, Ms. Palmer appeared confused about many aspects of this interview/examination throughout the interview/examination. She was not oriented to the year, the date, or the day; she was oriented to the month and the season. She was able to repeat three items and to recall two of them several minutes after. (This was on the MMSE administration.) She was not able to subtract serial sevens past 93, and her overall score on the MMSE of 19 was at the lowest possible number end of the "Mildly Impaired" range.

As mentioned above, Ms. Palmer was confused about her family, her present situation, and her husband; she was unrealistic, in my view, about her ability to take care of herself at home if her husband were to leave: "If the house were sold, what would you do?" "Move into an apartment." "Is the house sold?" "Yes, but I'll move in there anyhow."

After presenting and discussing some of Ms. Palmer's mental status findings, Dr. Harrison next gave examples of Ms. Palmer's own unusual, even bizarre, comments.

In a similar vein, Ms. Palmer insisted during this interview/examination that she "doesn't need nurse aid for 24 hours," and that in terms of ADLs (such as food preparation) she was similarly vague and unrealistic: "I'd eat out." She also expressed suspicious feelings about her present aide at Forest Hills, indicating that the aide "tried to steal everything," a feeling that she has had with her previous home health aides.

When Dr. Watkins and I briefly interviewed Ms. Palmer alone, she was unchanged in terms of her demeanor and presentation from how she had presented during the lengthy interview/examination prior to Ms. Burns' leaving. She told us, for example, that her "husband comes ever other day, every two days, once a week, I don't remember the last time."

In addition to these observations and discussion about Ms. Palmer's psychiatric/neuropsychiatric presentation, and comments about her physical frailty, I also noted a number of surgical scars on her legs, and in that context, noted her prior history of three operations for hip surgery (the original on her left, the second on her right, and a revision operation on her right, according to Ms. Burns).

Ms. Palmer's multiple medications have already been noted; the reader is referred to available records and materials for details.

Clinical Diagnostic Impressions

In keeping with the current diagnostic nomenclature and format of the *Diagnostic and Statistical Manual of Mental Disorders, Fourth Edition, Text Revision* (2000), or *DSM-IV-TR,* of the American Psychiatric Association, clinical diagnostic impressions for Ms. Palmer can be presented as follows:

Axis I (Clinical Disorders):

1. Dementia NOS [not otherwise specified], likely dementia of the Alzheimer's type, with late onset, complicated by chronic alcoholism.
2. Alcohol dependence, by history (reported by Ms. Burns), in institutional remission.

Axis II (Personality Disorders):

No Diagnosis.

Axis III (General Medical Conditions):

Ms. Palmer's multiple medical problems have already been described, including her Parkinsonism; her status post three hip surgery procedures; her hypertension; her GERD; as well as her cognitive impairment.

The reader is referred to applicable records and materials from Ms. Palmer's Forest Hills chart, described above and elsewhere in records and materials available for review in this matter, for further information and details.

Axis IV (Psychosocial and Environmental Problems):

Ms. Palmer's main present "Psychosocial and Environmental Problems" in my view pertain to her "Problems with primary support group" (her divorcing her husband and her strained relationship with her daughter, both of which are confusing to her because of her dementia), and her "Problems related to the social environment" (her likelihood of having to leave her family home following the divorce from her husband; her dislike of her present placement); "Housing Problems" (as just described); and the interactions of all these problem areas in an elderly cognitively impaired individual in poor physical and mental health, dependent on others for her day-to-day living, opinion applies here.

Axis V (Global Assessment of Functioning [GAF]):

A Global Assessment of Functioning (GAF) Scale score for Ms. Palmer of 40–50 signifying "serious symptoms . . . serious impairment in social, occupational, or school functioning . . . [to] . . . Some impairment in reality testing or communication . . . major impairment in several areas, such as work or school, family relations, judgment, thinking or mood" (language excerpted, in part, from the *DSM-IV-TR*, in my opinion, applies here).

Last, the evaluator's "Summary and Opinions" should be self-evident from the preceding sections of the report. In this case, those sections lead to the inevitable conclusion ("opinion") that Ms. Palmer is neither (and is not likely to become) "competent" or "not dangerous [for purposes of that aspect of this evaluation] to self or others." Nevertheless, both points should be made in a clear and explicit way, as they are in this report.

Summary and Opinions

Ms. Greta Palmer is a 92-year-old (DOB: December 18, XXXX) widowed and remarried (presently divorcing) white female, a former interior decorator by training and profession for many years (and retired for many years), currently placed at the Forest Hills facility (Bakertown), and presently involved, to my understanding, in a divorce action with her second husband as well as the present competency and civil commitment evaluation involving Dr. Reginald Watkins's and my clinical evaluation.

In addition to her personal and psychosocial background and history, Ms. Palmer has reportedly had a history for many years of chronic alcohol use, to the point of debilitation, according to her daughter. This left her in a situation in which her second husband (Charles Palmer, CPA; the couple was married in XXXX) has recently sued for divorce, resulting in complicated legal issues and activities, and bringing about the necessity, as I understand, for this present psychiatric/neuropsychiatric/addiction medicine competency evaluation of Ms. Palmer.

Ms. Palmer's background and history; the history of the events that led to this present competency evaluation; my psychiatric/neuropsychiatric/addiction medicine observations and findings concerning Ms. Palmer; and my clinical diagnostic impressions of Ms. Palmer are all as described above and elsewhere in records and materials available for review in this matter. That information will not be repeated in this section of this report.

By virtue of Ms. Palmer's background and history (likely complicated and aggravated by her chronic alcoholism); her present clinical presentation (as confused, and manifesting the cognitive loss and impairment described above); her inability to respond to practical questions about her ADLs (leading to the inference that she is not able to take care of herself, in my view); and noting the present difficult and stressful situation involving her husband's divorcing her, it is my psychiatric/neuropsychiatric/addiction medicine opinion—held with a degree of reasonable medical probability—that as of the time of my interview/examination of Ms. Palmer (on July 5, XXXX) and for at least the reasonable foreseeable future after that—if ever—Ms. Palmer is (and will be) unable to take care of herself from either a psychiatric/neuropsychiatric perspective or a medical/physical perspective, and that by virtue of the chronicity of the medical and psychiatric/neuropsychiatric conditions that have led to her present situation, as well as her lack of clinical improvement in a stable and supportive setting (specifically, Forest Hills) and her aging, she is not likely to improve clinically to the point of being considered competent to take care of herself and her affairs in the reasonably foreseeable future, if ever. That point renders her dangerous to self, according to applicable state law, as I understand that law. Ms. Palmer's irritability and periodic aggressiveness, in addition, make her likely dangerous to others in the reasonably foreseeable future, as she has been in the past.

> **After presenting her clinical opinions about the two areas to be addressed in this evaluation, Dr. Harrison, in effect, offered a disclaimer recognizing but supporting legal/court determinations about Ms. Palmer concerning the two issues in this matter.**

Recognizing that competency as such is a legal/court determination, and not a medical/psychiatric/clinical one, it is nevertheless my psychiatric/neuropsychiatric/addiction medicine opinion—held with a degree of reasonable medical probability—that inferences about Ms. Greta Palmer's underlying mental state and psychiatric/neuropsychiatric/addiction medicine condition as of the time of my interview/examination of her and for the reasonably foreseeable future after that *do* support a legal/court determination that Ms. Palmer is *not* generally competent as of the present, and will *not* be likely to be restored to such competency in the reasonably foreseeable future, if ever. It is also my professional opinion—held with a degree of reasonable medical probability—that these inferences make Ms. Palmer likely dangerous to herself and others at present and for the reasonably foreseeable future, also according to applicable state law, as I understand that law.

> **Last, Dr. Harrison wrote the customary disclaimers, distinguishing her forensic report from a purely clinical one.**

The referenced individual was examined with reference to specific circumstances emanating from the incident in question, in accordance with the restrictive rules concerning an independent medical examination. It is, therefore, understood that no treatment was given or suggested and that no doctor/patient relationship exists.

I aver that the information contained in this document was prepared by the undersigned and is the work of the undersigned. It is true to the best of my knowledge and information and has not been modified by anyone other than the undersigned.

Please do not hesitate to contact me if you have questions about this evaluation and report, or if you anticipate requiring additional services from me in connection with this matter.

Thank you very much.

Sincerely,

Regina Harrison, MD, MPH,

Diplomate, American Board of Psychiatry and Neurology (P)

Certified, American Society of Addiction Medicine

Case Analysis and Outcome

In evaluations of individuals for civil competency (which often occur in the context of guardianship or conservatorship proceedings), the evaluating mental health professional usually focuses on the evaluee's cognitive capacity to engage in general activities (such as taking care of oneself, shopping, cooking, cleaning, and so forth) and/or specific tasks (such as entering into contracts, making valid wills, and other such tasks), especially when that individual's cognitive ability to carry out such a task is questioned.

In this particular case, with a very dysfunctional background and history, and with both organic (dementia) and other (schizophrenia and substance abuse) psychiatric conditions in her history, the confluence of all of these factors in Ms. Palmer's case led to the inferences by the consulting mental health professionals (two, in this case) that she was not generally competent to take care of herself. That clinical impression, in turn, supported the assignment of a guardian for Ms. Palmer, although the specific issue of who would be the best guardian for her (which was not contested in this particular case) was not an issue to be addressed within the scope of this particular evaluation/consultation.

The attorney who is seeking professional mental health consultation/evaluation in matters such as this should be aware of the practical clinical distinction between what may be termed general and specific areas of competency, and should make that distinction clear to his/her consulting/evaluating mental health professional. Conversely, the mental health professional performing the consultation/evaluation should also be aware of this distinction, and should be specific with retaining counsel about the extent to which the consultation/evaluation responds to either or both of these areas.

Referring to the pointers in the expert/attorney and expert/court relationship, in this particular case, a prompt forensic evaluation was necessitated by the evaluee's deteriorating clinical condition. Dr. Harrison's rapid consultation and writing of her report, and close contact with retaining counsel, enabled the Competency and Commitment hearings for Ms. Palmer to take place quickly, without the necessity for Dr. Harrison to testify in person. Ms. Palmer was involuntarily committed to a local university-affiliated psychiatric hospital, received good treatment, and was doing well, as of Dr. Harrison's last contact with retaining counsel about Ms. Palmer.

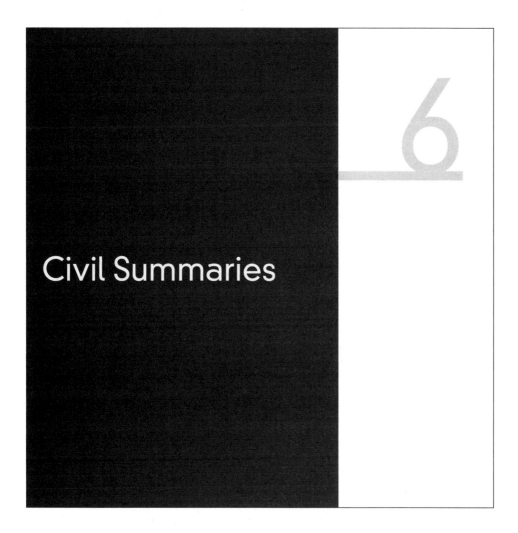

Civil Summaries

Similar to Chapter 4, in this chapter we present "Summary and Opinions" excerpts from a broader series of civil forensic mental health reports than is given in the four full reports from Chapter 5. We do this, as we did in Chapter 4, to enable the reader to learn about a wider variety of civil forensic mental health topics than space and time in this volume permit in the form of full reports.

As in Chapter 4, with a wide of variety of excerpted case examples, we convey to the reader a sense of the range and scope of civil matters in which forensic mental health evaluations and reports come into play.

Personal Injury

The plaintiff in this civil action was exposed to the World Trade Center attack on September 11, 2001, and alleged that significant psychological and physical trauma was sustained by that event. The plaintiff claimed further trauma caused by the employer in forcing a termination based on the sustained damages, resulting in an inability to return to the workplace in a meaningful position.

In the opinion of the forensic psychiatrist, the plaintiff's PTSD had abated by the time of this evaluation and, further, a return to gainful employment was both desired by the plaintiff and possible.

Personal Injury

The plaintiff in this civil action brought suit against a tour bus operator as a result of a slip and fall alleged to have occurred on the steps on the bus in which the plaintiff had been a passenger. Investigation disclosed that the plaintiff had been drinking to excess while a passenger. In addition, the plaintiff, an insulin-dependent diabetic, had not taken any prescribed medication for that illness any time during the day in which the accident took place. In the hospital emergency department where the plaintiff was taken after the accident, the blood sugar was elevated and blood alcohol level was above that associated with intoxication.

In the view of the forensic psychiatrist whose professional opinion was requested by the defendant, the plaintiff's consumption of alcohol together with the lack of prescribed medication for diabetic control both contributed to the accident.

Personal Injury

This case arose from a civil action brought by the victim of an automobile accident in which the plaintiff suffered serious multiple injuries and the adult child of the victim was killed.

It was the opinion of the forensic psychiatrist, based on a review of all relevant and available records and a face-to-face meeting, the plaintiff was experiencing a clinically significant degree of depression resulting from the child's death, along with guilt feelings arising from the inability to avoid the accident.

Employment Law

The individual in this case claimed to have been the victim of a variety of deliberate and adverse workplace actions that ultimately led to a compelled resignation and, subsequently, to a lawsuit. As a result of the workplace allegations, the plaintiff was treated by a number of psychiatrists, one of whom provided the opinion that the plaintiff was suffering from PTSD.

In the opinion of the forensic psychiatrist, however, the plaintiff's perceptions of workplace problems did not clinically meet the requirements for a PTSD diagnosis. However, it was noted that there was mild-to-moderate impairment and symptomatology; that it was the plaintiff's perception that such symptomatology was workplace- related; and that there were other (non-workplace claim–related) stressors present, all of which have added to and worsened that symptomatology.

Personal Injury

The underlying issues in this case concerned the individual's psychotic conditions and relevant treatment and pharmacotherapy. The individual's medical/psychiatric problems were the result of a motor vehicle accident that had caused medical/psychiatric issues and prevented employment. At the time of the report the individual was undergoing medical and psychiatric treatment and was being administered Imitrex, trazodone, and Seroquel to reduce anxiety and depression.

Based on available records and a face-to-face meeting, it was the opinion of the forensic psychiatrist that the then-ongoing treatments and medications should be continued with a goal of rehabilitation and return to active employment.

Employment Law

The individual was employed for several years as an education professional. Subsequent to requiring breast surgery with attendant chemotherapy and radiology treatments, the individual became increasingly withdrawn and exhibited behaviors in the workplace that were troubling to the employer.

It was the opinion of the forensic psychiatrist, whose professional help was requested by the employer, that the individual posed no danger in the workplace. Further, the psychiatrist recommended a number of other steps that included transfer to another location, a more stable work schedule, a change in medication, a program of moderate exercise, and psychotherapy.

Employment Law

The individual in this case was the victim of workplace problems that finally caused involuntary resignation. As a result of that experience, the individual became upset, worried, depressed, agitated, and angry, conditions that led to psychiatric treatment and pharmacotherapy. In addition, physical issues arose (to include elevated cholesterol caused by an antidepressant medication).

In the opinion of the forensic psychiatrist, and after a review of relevant records and a face-to-face meeting, the individual suffered from adjustment disorder with depressed mood, chronic, that caused impairment and was created by the employment experience.

Employment Law

The individual in this case alleged unfair and unacceptable treatment in the workplace and filed a lawsuit against the employer. It was the claim of the individual that the treatment received, and which was the basis for the lawsuit, had created severe depression that made subsequent employment impossible.

In the opinion of the forensic psychiatrist, this individual's case, while not strictly satisfying the clinical requirement of posttraumatic stress disorder, did present a clinical picture similar to it, including recurrent and intrusive recollections of the event; recurrent dreams of the event; acting or feeling as though the event was recurring; persistent avoidance of stimuli associated with the trauma; hypervigilance; difficulty in concentrating; and irritability. Further, it was the psychiatrist's opinion that the workplace experiences had "spoiled" the individual's chances for success in future employment at the very least for the then-reasonably foreseeable future.

Malpractice

The plaintiff in this lawsuit was pushed into the path of an oncoming bus by an individual who was a diagnosed paranoid schizophrenic, had a history of violence, and was not taking prescribed medications. The plaintiff suffered severe injuries and filed suit against a number of hospitals, individuals, and government agencies.

Despite being treated by two health care providers just before the assault upon the plaintiff and while observed by those providers, the attacker apparently displayed bizarre, psychotic, paranoid, and potentially dangerous ideas and comments, points that were of particular importance given the attacker's history of the long-standing paranoid psychiatric disorder, which was known to the providers. There was no communication between the providers regarding the individual's dangerous potential. In the opinion of the forensic psychiatrist, these providers deviated from accepted standards of medical/psychiatric care by that lack of communication and by taking no action to restrain or involuntarily hospitalize the attacker.

Malpractice (Nursing Home)

The defendant in this case was a nursing home. An elderly resident of the facility died and was buried without notification to the next-of-kin of either event. The next-of-kin, and plaintiff in this civil action, was described as being angry and upset about the incident and subsequently sought and received counseling and psychiatric care. It was felt necessary to obtain an opinion of a forensic psychiatrist as to the plaintiff's mental condition relevant to the incident. In the opinion of the forensic psychiatrist, the plaintiff's mental condition was improving with the greatest stressor being the continuing litigation.

Malpractice (Rehabilitation Facility)

This case involved a lawsuit brought by an employee of the defendant, a rehabilitation facility, who was sexually assaulted by a patient. The assault occurred after the offender was transferred to another facility and came under the care of the plaintiff. In the view of the plaintiff it was the duty of the defendant to advise of the possibility that the patient represented a potential threat as a sex offender.

In the opinion of the forensic psychiatrist, there was no reasonable way for the facility to have predicted such potential behavior and there was also a question as to whether it could have provided information about a mental state relevant to possible sex offender behavior without violating confidentiality guidelines.

Dram Shop Liability

This case concerned a lawsuit brought by the estate of an individual who became intoxicated while a bar patron and who, while visibly intoxicated, was served alcohol. After leaving the bar, the individual was stopped by a police officer while operating a motor vehicle. A confrontation took place in which the individual assaulted the officer, attempted to take the officer's weapon, and was fatally shot. Suit was filed against the bar seeking damages on the basis of dram shop liability.

It was the opinion of the psychiatrist retained by the estate and based on an examination of available records, that given the decedent's history of violence and aggression—including such behavior while drinking—that decedent's behavior was an inevitable consequence of his being served at the bar while already visibly intoxicated.

Sexually Violent Predator

The issue in this case was whether the adjudicated sex offender presented, at that time or in the then-reasonably foreseeable future, a "highly likely" risk of sexual reoffending if placed in a less secure facility for continuing treatment.

The individual, prior to this evaluation, had a cerebrovascular accident (CVA; stroke) and myocardial infarction (MI) and had very limited mobility, being unable to ambulate without assistance. Based on these physical considerations along with physiologic and psychological factors pertaining to reduced libido and sexuality, the opinion of the forensic psychiatrist was that the individual was "highly unlikely" to reoffend if transferred to a less secure setting.

Civil Commitment/Competency

This individual is described as mildly mentally retarded and having a history of serious psychiatric disorders that were identified in early childhood. Following an incident of alleged sexual abuse of a child, the individual was found incompetent to stand trial for the offense and was civilly committed to a mental institution. The opinion of a forensic psychiatrist was deemed necessary relevant to the possibility of this individual being released and treated as an outpatient.

Based on the individual's inpatient history, that is, passive, isolative, and demonstrating no aggressive or dangerous behavior, or sexually offensive behaviors, it was the opinion of the forensic psychiatrist that this individual could be safely discharged to family members.

Sexually Violent Predator

Following conviction for several self-reported sex offenses, this individual was incarcerated for two decades between prison and a sex offender unit. The issue was whether there was a "highly likely" chance of reoffending if the individual was placed in a less structured and secure facility.

Following a review of all relevant records and conducting a face-to-face interview/examination, it was the opinion of the forensic psychiatrist that it was not "highly likely" that this individual would reoffend sexually. Among the factors considered in arriving at this opinion were that the individual had not been a user of illicit drugs for over a decade, had undergone substance abuse treatment and wished to continue it, and had apparently benefited from continuing psychiatric and sex-offender specific treatment. It was, however, the recommendation of the forensic psychiatrist that this individual not be immediately released to a less secure setting given the lack of exposure to the outside community for many years and that, instead, the release be more graduated, allowing the individual to incrementally become accustomed to outside life.

Sexually Violent Predator (NGRI)

This individual had been adjudicated NGRI of a sex offense charge. The history of psychiatric illness is extensive and includes bipolar disorder and two psychiatric hospitalizations prior to that resulting from the NGRI determination. The individual claimed no knowledge of the sex offense and experienced only limited treatment success while in a secure treatment facility. During such commitment the individual was engaged in inappropriate behavior with staff members and failed to comply with the medication regimen.

It was the opinion of the forensic psychiatrist that this individual presented a probable risk for dangerous hostile behaviors for the then-foreseeable future. It was recommended that pharmacotherapy be closely monitored and, further, that counseling psychotherapy be provided as part of overall treatment, the latter being necessary because of bizarre ideas noted during a face-to-face interview. A transfer to a less secure environment was not recommended.

Caveat Proceeding

This caveat proceeding was brought by individuals who had been the principal beneficiaries under a will executed by the deceased testator. A subsequent will named a new beneficiary and provided significantly reduced asset distributions to the individuals who had been designated in the first will. The second will was thus challenged on the grounds that, first, the testator was not competent when the second will was executed and, second, that the testator, who was terminally ill and facing imminent death, had been subjected to undue influence on the part of a long-time family servant. The servant was the principal beneficiary under the second will.

In the professional opinion of the forensic psychiatrist retained by the beneficiaries under the first will, based on a review of relevant and available medical records and the reported behavior of the testator before her death, including her relationship with the new beneficiary, and despite the many illnesses suffered by the testator, the second will appeared valid. Among the documents reviewed by the psychiatrist were opinions offered by the testator's primary care physician, pleadings, depositions, and interrogatories.

Sexually Violent Predator

This case involves a convicted sexually violent predator with a criminal history that includes other types of offenses. The individual also has a history of substance abuse, depression, and emotional suffering caused by abandonment, physical abuse, and sexual abuse. During the course of custodial treatment (prior to a commitment hearing), this individual was generally described as making satisfactory clinical progress. A forensic psychiatrist reviewed all available and relevant documents and conducted an interview. In the opinion of the forensic psychiatrist, there were several factors that would point to release on an outpatient basis to the community under a Megan's Law supervision program. These factors include inpatient treatment progress, and close friends available to provide necessary emotional support.

Sexually Violent Predator

This individual, a convicted sex offender, had been confined to penal and mental institutions throughout much of adulthood. When the sentence for the most recent sexual offense was almost completed, a hearing was held that classified the individual as a sex offender under the provisions of the law. It was later questioned as to whether the lack of expert psychiatric testimony at the hearing resulted in a different outcome from a hearing at which expert psychiatric testimony were present. The question of competency to stand trial was also raised because of the individual's stated desire for postconviction relief.

In the opinion of the forensic psychiatrist in this case, the lack of testimony regarding the classification as a "repetitive and compulsive" sex offender would not have had any impact on the determination made at the hearing. It was also the opinion of the forensic psychiatrist that the individual was competent to stand trial, some of the factors behind that conclusion being the level of anger and resistance exhibited, the demonstrated lack of cooperation, and the denial of any wrongdoing concerning the offense charged.

Toxic Exposure

While employed by a medical facility, this individual, with a previously undistinguished medical history, was exposed to a highly toxic substance that resulted in claimed severe and complicated medical issues to include infectious disease and substance abuse that prevented a return to work. The individual filed a lawsuit against the employer and the opinion of a forensic psychiatrist was deemed necessary.

In the opinion of the forensic psychiatrist, based on a review of all relevant medical records and subject interviews, a return to work was not only possible but advisable, and further that the motivation of the individual appeared to be that of "secondary gain," that is, a need for attention, vindication, and financial reward.

Professional Regulation

The attorney in this case voluntarily discontinued his successful and stress-filled practice of law after experiencing depression and feeling unable to carry out those duties required in his practice. Soon after the discontinuance of the practice, numerous complaints were filed regarding the attorney's actions. One major concern was whether the attorney had the ability to participate with counsel in mounting and maintaining a defense to the complaints. A second was whether the individual could return to a practice of law.

It was the opinion of the forensic psychiatrist, based on an examination and interview of the individual, that the attorney possessed the necessary cognitive and emotional ability to participate with counsel and, further, that the attorney possessed the necessary cognitive and emotional ability to practice law, albeit with a reduced caseload and in a less stressful practice area.

Divorce: BWS/PTSD

The issue here revolved around the claims of the wife that she was a battered woman (BWS) and suffering from PTSD. The marital relationship could be described as having been, at the very least, highly contentious with allegations of mental and physical abuse. The latter claims were unsubstantiated.

The opinion of the forensic psychiatrist in the case was based on a review of all relevant records and intensive face-to-face interviews with both parties to the divorce action. As a result of these examinations it was the opinion of the forensic psychiatrist that the wife failed to meet the BWS criteria and that the husband did not clinically present as a batterer. Further, in the opinion of the psychiatrist, the wife failed to meet the diagnostic criteria for PTSD.

Contract Duress

The question presented in this civil action brought by the plaintiff (an adult son) against his father was whether the plaintiff had been under extreme duress when he executed a document giving the father a large percentage of a legal settlement awarded to the son, who at the time of the settlement was a minor.

It was the opinion of the forensic psychiatrist that the plaintiff was not competent to execute the document in question, such lack of competence being based on a number of factors. Among other points noted in the psychiatrist's opinion was that the father had been manipulative of his son, particularly regarding the legal settlement, for many years, with threats to provide information that would show that the settlement had been obtained through fraud. The threat was an empty one, although details of the settlement might have proved embarrassing. The relationship that developed was one not based on any high degree of trust on the part of the son toward the father. Finally, the opinion continued with the point that the father's insistence on having a share of the settlement, along with all other elements in the father-son relationship, culminated in a feeling on the part of the son that he should sign the document even after his stated belief, once having done so, that it was the wrong thing to do.

Conclusion

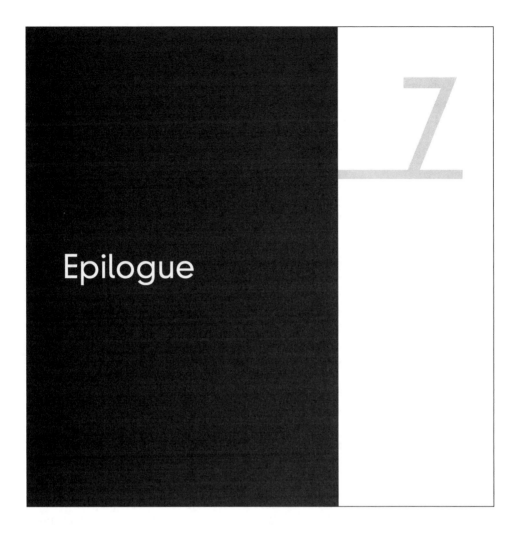

Epilogue

In this book, we have presented one particular format for forensic mental health reports, with numerous full redacted examples using that format, and a series of summaries of those examples that illustrate some of the wide variety of areas and topics addressed. We have provided commentary and discussion of some of these cases, in order to relate the legal issues in these evaluations—the forensic mental health questions raised by retaining counsel or the court—to the clinically based reports about the mental health professional's findings, impressions, and opinions concerning those issues.

We have not attempted here to write an encyclopedic reference handbook of forensic mental health practice. However, by reviewing the cases and commentary presented in tandem with the background and theory in any of a number of forensic mental health textbooks and monographs, articles, and Internet sources (such as those listed in Appendices B1–B4), the reader will achieve a practical view of the myriad ways in which mental health professionals may consult in the forensic arena.

Here we return to the list of pointers, which we believe will be of value to mental health practitioners in their forensic work. If dutifully followed, these pointers (which are essentially a mixture of common sense and courtesy, along with professionalism) will greatly assist in making the interaction, cooperation, and communication among mental health professionals, retaining counsel, and others more harmonious and efficient.

At numerous and relevant times in the text, particularly in the case commentaries, we have referred to these points. It was our belief that repeating and expanding upon them here would be of value.

- *Maintain contact with other professionals involved in the case.* In our experience, it is rarely true that "too many cooks spoil the broth." Ongoing professional cooperation and communication are always a plus.
- *Always be ready to listen to other views.* Nobody has a monopoly on knowledge. The acquisition of knowledge and new and different perspectives, and the vetting of new ideas, are all activities to be encouraged between experts and retaining counsel and the courts.
- *Be attentive. Focus on the subject at hand.* Despite the modern interest in multitasking, its value is not always practical or professional. For the forensic mental health practitioner, there must be only one point of focus, that being the individual(s) being evaluated, and the forensic mental health issues raised in that evaluation.
- *Avoid unnecessary delays and take responsibility for them if they occur.* Appointments must be kept on time, reports provided with care and diligence, and all other responsibilities fulfilled. But, bad things do happen: When they do, admit to them, and learn from them.
- *Communicate clearly. Avoid clouding of communication with needless professional jargon.* Think about how your communication will be received and perceived by the intended audience, even if that audience is only one person. Make messages simple with as little room as possible for misunderstanding and obfuscation.
- *Return telephone calls and related communications promptly.* You must assume that when someone calls you, e-mails you, or otherwise communicates with you, that person believes it was important and necessary to do so. Within reason, close the communications gap and return the call as soon as possible. If a particular mode of communication is not to your liking (such as e-mail), make your communication preference clear to others at the beginning of your professional relationship, and also try to accommodate your communicator's preference as well.
- *Time is precious. Don't waste it.* Time management is a skill that comes more easily to some than to others. Wasting time costs resources: your own and those of others in the professional community. Spend some time learning to manage it.

The efforts we have expended on the preparation of this book were necessary to illustrate the growing need for effective forensic report writing in the mental health professions.

We caution our readers that it requires more than a cursory examination of such a book as this to successfully fill the need for these reports. The kind of reports set out in these pages cannot be hastily created and then allowed to fend for themselves in an environment where their use is critical. Care must be taken in the preparation of all forensic reports, surely not the least being those in the mental health area. And, further, the writer must always be conscious of the intended reader audience, as is the case with any written document. Judges, lawyers, other mental health professionals, social workers, and others form part of the audience that may need to be not only informed but, indeed, persuaded by the contents of the document.

Finally, of course, the reports in both content and appearance are representative of the writer's knowledge and professionalism.

In the final analysis, in the same way that an attorney's "time is his stock in trade" (attributed to Abraham Lincoln, 1860), the forensic mental health professional's written report of findings, impressions, and opinions may represent the most important part of that individual's practice. For negotiation by counsel; as a record of materials reviewed and of the multiple parts of the consultant's evaluation (analogous to an attorney's trial notebook); as a document both in forming the forensic mental health professional's expert opinion in live, video-taped, audiotaped, or telephonic testimony; and in forming the basis for direct testimony and cross-examination testimony of the expert, the importance of the forensic mental health professional's written report cannot be underestimated.

By presenting a practical how-to handbook for writing persuasive, compelling, and well-organized reports, we hope to reduce the fear and apprehension of "all ye who enter here"—the often anxiety-provoking world of forensic mental health practice—and to make that practice a bit easier for all concerned: mental health professionals, legal and court professionals, and the many others involved in the American justice system.

Appendix A

GLOSSARY: KEY ACRONYMS FOR MENTAL HEALTH PROFESSIONALS

For the convenience of readers, the authors have provided this glossary of acronyms used in this book.

AD/HD	Attention Deficit/Hyperactivity Disorder
ADL	Activities of Daily Living
AUDIT	Alcohol Use Disorders Identification Test
BAC	Blood Alcohol Concentration
BAC	Blood Alcohol Content
BDI-II	Beck Depression Inventory, 2nd edition
BWS	Battered Woman Syndrome
CCSE	Cognitive Capacity Screening Examination
CST	Competency to Stand Trial
CVA	Cerebrovascular Accident (stroke)
DAST	Drug Abuse Screening Test
DSM-IV-TR	*Diagnostic and Statistical Manual of Mental Disorders, Fourth Edition, Text Revision*
DUI	Driving Under the Influence
GAF	Global Assessment of Functioning
GSW	Gunshot Wound
LOP	Level of Privileges
MAST	Michigan Alcohol Screening Test
MCMI-III	Millon Clinical Multiaxial Inventory, 3rd edition
MI	Myocardial Infarction (heart attack)
MMPI	Minnesota Multiphasic Personality Inventory, 2nd edition
MMSE	Mini-Mental State Examination
NGRI (or NGI)	Not Guilty by Reason of Insanity (depending on jurisdiction usage)
PTSD	Posttraumatic Stress Disorder
SDP	Sexually Dangerous Person
SVP	Sexually Violent Predator

Appendix B1

SELECTED LIST OF BOOKS AND MONOGRAPHS FOR WRITING FORENSIC MENTAL HEALTH REPORTS AND EVALUATIONS

Over about the past 10 years, publication of books about forensic psychology, psychiatry, and other mental health sciences has burgeoned, both in specific and specialized volumes and in encyclopedic tomes. The array of such publications may appear bewildering to newcomers to the field, in their efforts to do clinically based forensic psychiatric/psychological evaluations and to embody these evaluations in a written report.

What follows is a selected list of those books and monographs that have been helpful to the authors in their work in writing reports of forensic psychiatric evaluations and in researching numerous topics for publication and teaching in various areas in forensic psychiatry and psychology.

This list is by no means exhaustive. The interested reader may also consult applicable Web sites (Appendix B3) for additional information about books and monographs published in these fields.

Alexander, G. J., & Scheflin, A. W. (Eds.). (1998). *Law and mental disorder.* Durham, NC: Carolina Academic Press.

Arrigo, B. A., & Shipley, S. L. (2005). Introduction to *Forensic psychology: Issues and controversies in law, law enforcement and corrections* (2nd ed.). New York: Elsevier Academic Press.

Babitsky, S., Mangraviti, J. J., & Melhorn, J. M. (2004). *Writing and defending your IME report: The comprehensive guide.* Falmouth, MA: SEAK.

Bradford, J. M. W. (Ed.). (1992, September). Clinical forensic psychiatry. *The Psychiatric Clinics of North America, 15*(3), ii-741.

Bursten, B. (2001). *Psychiatry on trial: Fact and fantasy in the courtroom.* Jefferson, NC: McFarland.

Curran, W. J., McGarry, A. L., & Shah, S. A. (1986). *Forensic psychiatry and psychology.* Philadelphia: F. D. David.

Dershowitz, A. M. (1994). *The abuse excuse and other cop-outs, sob stories, and evasions of responsibility.* Boston: Little, Brown.

Dorran, P. B. (1982). *The expert witness.* Washington, DC: Planners Press.

Dupont, R. L. (Ed.). (2000). *Forensic issues in addiction medicine.* Chevy Chase, MD: American Society of Addiction Medicine.

Faust, D., Ziskin, J., & Hiers, J. B. (1991). *Brain damage claims: Coping with neuropsychological evidence.* Los Angeles: Law and Psychology Press.

Geiselman, R. E. (1996). *Eyewitness expert testimony: Handbook for the forensic psychiatrist, psychologist and attorney* (2nd ed.). Balboa Island, CA: ACFP Press.

Geiselman, R. E. (Ed.). (2004). *Psychology of murder: Readings in forensic science.* Balboa Island, CA: ACFP Press.

Godwin, G. M. (Ed.). (2001). *Criminal psychology and forensic technology: A collaborative approach to effective profiling.* Boca Raton, FL: CRC Press.

Gold, L. H. (2004). *Sexual harassment: Psychiatric assessment in employment litigation.* Washington, DC: American Psychiatric Publishing.

Greenfield, D. P. (1995). *Prescription drug abuse and dependence: How prescription drug abuse contributes to the drug abuse epidemic.* Springfield, IL: Charles C. Thomas.

Gunn, J., & Taylor, P. J. (Eds.). (1993). *Forensic psychiatry: Clinical, legal and ethical issues.* London: Butterworth Heinemann.

Gutheil, T. G., & Applebaum, P. S. (2005). *Clinical handbook of psychiatry and the law* (4th ed.). Baltimore, MD: Lippincott, Williams & Wilkins.

Gutheil, T. G., & Simon, R. I. (2002). *Mastering forensic psychiatric practice: Advanced strategies for the expert witness.* Washington, DC: American Psychiatric Publishing.

Insanity Defense Work Group. (1984). *Issues in forensic psychiatry.* Washington, DC: American Psychiatric Press.

Katz, J., Goldstein, J., & Dershowitz, A. M. (1967). *Psychoanalysis, psychiatry and law.* New York: The Free Press.

McDonald, J. J., & Kulick, F. P. (Eds.). (2001). *Mental and emotional injuries in employment litigation* (2nd ed., with 2006 Supplement). Washington, DC: BNA Press.

Melton, G. B., Petrila, J., Poythress, N. G., & Slobogin, C. (1997). *Psychological evaluations for the courts: A handbook for mental health professionals and lawyers* (2nd ed.). New York: The Guilford Press.

Monahan, J., Steadman, H. J., et al. (2001). *Rethinking risk assessment: The Macarthur study of mental disorder and violence.* New York: Oxford University Press.

Moran, R. (Ed.). (1985, February). The insanity defense. *The Annals of the American Academy of Political and Social Science, 477,* 9–190.

Perlin, M. L. (1999). *Mental disability law: Cases and materials.* Durham, NC: Carolina Academic Press.

Price, D. R., & Lees-Haley, P. R. (Eds.). (1995). *The insurer's handbook of psychological injury claims.* Seattle, WA: Claims Books.

Resnick, P. J. (Ed.). (1999). Forensic psychiatry. *The Psychiatric Clinics of North America, 22*(1), 1–219.

Rogers, R., & Shuman, D. W. (2005). *Fundamentals of forensic practice: Mental health and criminal law.* New York: Springer Science and Business Media.

Rosner, R. (Ed.). (2003). *Principles and practice of forensic psychiatry* (2nd ed.). London: Arnold.

Sadoff, R. L. (1975). *Forensic psychiatry: A practical guide for lawyers and psychiatrists.* Springfield, IL: Charles C. Thomas.

Sadoff, R. L. (Ed.). (1983, December). Forensic psychiatry. *The Psychiatric Clinics of North America, 6*(4), 1–783.

Schetky, D. H., & Benedek, E. T. (Eds.). (2002). *Principles and practice of child and adolescent forensic psychiatry.* Washington, DC: American Psychiatric Publishing.

Schlesinger, L. B. (Ed.). (2000). *Serial offenders: Current thought, recent findings.* Boca Raton, FL: CRC Press.

Shuman, D. W. (1986). *Psychiatric and psychological evidence.* New York: McGraw-Hill.

Simon, R. I. (2001). *Concise guide to clinical psychiatry and the law* (3rd ed.). Washington, DC: American Psychiatric Publishing.

Simon, R. I. (Ed.). (2003). *Posttraumatic stress disorder in litigation: Guidelines for forensic assessment* (2nd ed.). Washington, DC: American Psychiatric Publishing.

Simon, R. I., & Gold, L. H. (2004). *Textbook of forensic psychiatry.* Washington, DC: American Psychiatric Publishing.

Simon, R. I., & Shuman, D. W. (Eds.). (2002). *Retrospective assessment of mental states in litigation: Predicting the past.* Washington, DC: American Psychiatric Publishing.

Slovenko, R. (1998). *Psychotherapy and confidentiality: Testimonial privileged communication, breach of confidentiality, and reporting duties.* Springfield, IL: Charles C. Thomas.

Slovenko, R. (2002). *Law in psychiatry, psychiatry in law.* New York: Brunner-Rutledge.

Spring, R. L., Lacoursiere, R. B., & Weissenberger, G. (1989). *Patients, psychiatrists and lawyers: Law and the mental health system* (1991 Supplement). Cincinnati: Anderson.

Stone, A. A. (1975). *Mental health and law: A system in transition.* Rockville, MD: National Institutes of Mental Health.

Thenor, F. (2004). *Civil and criminal mental health law: A companion reference for forensic experts and attorneys. The essential cases.* Balboa Island, CA: ACFP Press.

Wrightsman, L. S. (2001). *Forensic psychology.* Stamford, CT: Wadsworth Thomson Learning.

Wrightsman, L. S., Nietzel, M. T., & Fortune, W. H. (1998). *Psychology and the legal system* (4th ed.). Pacific Grove, CA: Brooks/Cole.

Wulach, J. S. (1998). *Law and mental health professionals: New Jersey* (2nd ed.). Washington, DC: American Psychological Association.

Ziskin, J., & Faust, D. (1988). *Coping with psychiatric and psychological testimony* (4th ed.). Los Angeles: Law and Psychology Press.

Appendix B2

JOURNALS AND PERIODICALS OF LEGAL AND MENTAL HEALTH TOPICS FOR WRITING FORENSIC MENTAL HEALTH REPORTS

The professional literature in psychiatry, psychology, other mental health sciences, sociology, criminology, and the law is replete with journals, both general and specific, that deal with the broad topic of forensic psychiatry.

The following selective list of some general and some crossover (specifically dealing with legal and mental health topics) journals includes those that have been particularly helpful to the authors in their work in writing reports of forensic psychiatric evaluations and in researching topics for publications and teaching in various areas in forensic psychiatry, psychology, and law.

This list is by no means exhaustive. The interested reader may also consult applicable Web sites (Appendix B3) for additional information about journal publications in these fields.

- *American Journal of Forensic Psychiatry*
- *American Journal of Forensic Psychology*
- *American Journal of Psychiatry* (official journal of the American Psychiatric Association)
- *American Psychologist* (official journal of the American Psychological Association)
- *Behavioral Science and the Law*
- *British Journal of Psychiatry* (official journal of the British Psychiatric Association)
- *British Journal of Psychology* (official journal of the British Psychological Association)
- *British Journal of Psychological Medicine*
- *Journal of the American Academy of Psychiatry and Law*
- *Journal of Forensic Psychiatry* (British)
- *Journal of Forensic Sciences* (multidisciplinary, with periodic forensic psychiatry articles; the official journal of the American Association of Forensic Sciences)
- *Journal of Psychiatry and Law*
- *Law and Human Behavior*
- *The Neurolaw Letter* (a newsletter)

Appendix B3

INTERNET RESOURCES FOR THE MENTAL HEALTH PROFESSIONAL

A third source of information about forensic mental health topics and issues, the Internet, abounds with hundreds of entries, titles, and links to other sites. Many of these sources can be useful to the readers of this book in research for cases, reports, and writing projects.

However, as with any such use of the Internet, the reliability of Internet sources may be questionable. An Internet source may not be peer-reviewed or widely accepted, and may even be the idiosyncratic brainchild of the site's author(s). See, for example, Andrew Keen, *The Cult of the Amateur: How Today's Internet Is Killing Our Culture* (New York: Doubleday, 2007).

The user of the Internet for these purposes should be aware of this *caveat.* In our experience, the most useful Web sources in these areas, generally, are those with academic affiliations (such as universities and law schools), governmental sites, sites affiliated with published works in the field, and other such sites analogous to peer-reviewed or juried works in the printed media.

With the cautions just described, Appendix B3 gives a list of numerous Web sites concerning forensic mental health and legal topics and issues, which may be useful to the readers of this book.

- Academy of Behavioral Profiling [ABP]: www.profiling.org
- American Academy of Forensic Psychology: www.abfp.com
- American Academy of Psychiatry and the Law: www.aapl.org
- American College of Forensic Examiners: www.acfe.com
- American College of Forensic Psychiatry: www.forensicpsychiatry.cc
- American Journal of Forensic Psychiatry: www.forensicpsychonline.com/jrnl.htm
- American Psychiatric Association: www.psych.org
- American Psychological Association: www.apa.org
- American Psychological Association/Ethical Principles for Psychologists: www.apa.org/ethics/code2002.pdf
- American Psychology-Law Society [AP-LS]: www.ap-ls.org
- American Society of Criminology: www.asc41.com
- Anuario de Psicología Jurídica: www.copmadrid.org/publicaciones/juridica/juridica.htm
- Australian and New Zealand Journal of Criminology: www.ingentaconnect.com/content/aap/anzjc;jsessionid = rvuc9dhq2g6e.alice

Adapted and excerpted from: www.umdnj.edu/psyevnts/forensic.html

- Bazelon Center for Mental Health Law: www.bazelon.org
- Behavioral Sciences and the Law: www3.interscience.wiley.com/cgi-bin/jhome/3512?CRETRY = 1&SRETRY = 0
- British Journal of Criminology: bjc.oxfordjournals.org
- Canadian Journal of Criminology: www.ccja-acjp.ca/en/cjc.html
- Canadian Journal of Law and Society: www.rcds-cjls.uqam.ca/index_en.htm#a
- Canadian Law and Society Association: www.rcds-cjls.uqam.ca/index_en.htm
- Carpenter's Forensic Science Resources: www.tncrimlaw.com/forensic/f_psych.html
- Child Abuse and Neglect: www.elsevier.com/wps/find/journaldescription.cws_home/586/description
- Child Abuse Review: www3.interscience.wiley.com/cgi-bin/jhome/5060
- Children and Society: www3.interscience.wiley.com/cgi-bin/jhome/4805
- Crime and Delinquency: cad.sagepub.com
- Criminal Behaviour and Mental Health: www3.interscience.wiley.com/cgi-bin/jhome/112094296
- Criminal Justice and Behavior: cjb.sagepub.com
- Criminal Justice Links, including a section on juvenile delinquency sites: www.criminology.fsu.edu/p/cjl-main.php
- Criminologia.it, journal on the theory and science of criminology: www.criminologia.it
- Criminologia.org, Telematic Journal of Clinical Criminology: www.criminologia.org/rivista/rivista_cronaca.htm
- Criminologie: www.erudit.org/revue/crimino
- Criminology: An Interdisciplinary Journal: www.asc41.com/publications.html
- *Derecho Medico* by Julio César Galán Cortés, with information on Spanish law regarding malpractice and medical responsibility as well as forums on HIV, confidentiality, informed consent, etc.: www.terra.es/personal/jcgalan
- Ethical Guidelines for the Practice of Forensic Psychiatry: www.aapl.org/pdf/ETHICSGDLNS.pdf
- European Association of Psychology and Law [EAPL]: www.law.kuleuven.ac.be/eapl
- Findlaw Internet Legal Resources, including Law Crawler and directory of government officials: www.findlaw.com
- Forensic Psychiatry Site of Harold J. Bursztajn, MD: www.forensic-psych.com
- Forensic Psychology and Psychiatry Links of David Willshire: members.optusnet.com.au/dwillsh
- Forensische Psychiatrie und Psychotherapie: www.wsfpp-forensik.de
- Forenzic.com: www.forenzic.com
- Institute of Law, Psychiatry and Public Policy, at the University of Virginia: www.ilppp.virginia.edu
- The Institute of Mental Health Law specializes in all aspects of the British Mental Health Act of 1983: www.imhl.com
- International Academy of Law and Mental Health [IALMH]: www.ialmh.org

- International Association of Forensic Mental Health Services [IAFMHS]: www.iafmhs.org
- International Association for Forensic Psychotherapy [IAFP]: forensic psychotherapy.com
- The Journal of Credibility Assessment and Witness Psychology: truth. boisestate.edu/jcaawp/default.html
- Law and Psychology Review, the annual journal of the University of Alabama School of Law: www.law.ua.edu/lawpsychology
- Law and Society Association [LSA]: www.lawandsociety.org/
- Law and Society Review: www.lawandsociety.org/review.htm
- National Organization of Forensic Social Work [NOFSW]: www.nofsw. org
- Página Forense: www.arrakis.es/~jacoello/inicial.html
- Psicologia Giustizia: www.psicologiagiuridica.com
- PsyBar, LLC, a national professional services company offering psychological and psychiatric experts to law firms, courts, corporations, insurance companies, and government agencies: www.psybar.com
- Psychiatry and Law Updates by William H. Reid, MD, MPH, an educational and communication service for professionals, with commentary on recent developments and links to resources: www.reidpsychiatry.com
- Reddy's Forensic Page, large compilation of links on various forensic topics: www.forensicpage.com
- Rominger Legal has a comprehensive set of links to federal and state resources, organizations, professional directories and law categories, such as divorce, criminal, bankruptcy, etc.: www.romingerlegal.com
- Zeno's Forensic Site, with special section on psychiatry and psychology: www.forensic.to/forensic.html

Appendix B4

REFERENCES AND ARTICLES REGARDING FORENSIC MENTAL HEALTH REPORTS

Recognizing that "there's more than one way to skin a cat," what follows is a list of articles and chapters about formulating and writing forensic psychiatric and psychological reports. These materials have been particularly useful to the first author of this book, Daniel P. Greenfield, MD, MPH, MS, in his forensic report writing over the years.

Different approaches, styles, and formats are discussed in some of these pieces. In the final analysis, however, all agree that forensic reports for the legal system are clinically based and clinically informed, and are not legal documents.

Brakel, S. J. (1992, July). Legal tips for writing the psychological report in child custody and visitation cases. *Psychiatric Annals, 22*(7), 387–395.

Garrick, T. R., & Stotland, N. L. (1982, July). How to write a psychiatric consultation. *American Journal of Psychiatry, 139*(7), 849–855.

Gutheil, T. G. (1998). Writing to and for the legal system. In T. G. Gutheil, *The psychiatrist as expert witness* (chapter 8, pp. 101–110). Washington, DC: American Psychiatric Press.

Hoffman, B. H. (1986, February). How to write a psychiatric report for litigation following a personal injury. *American Journal of Psychiatry, 143*(2), 164–169.

Melton, C. B., Petrila, J., Poythress, N. G., & Slobogin, C. (1997). Report writing. In C. B. Melton et al., *Psychological evaluations for the courts* (2nd ed., section 18.03, pp. 523–527). New York: The Guilford Press.

Morrant, J. C. A. (1982, October 15). Family practice: How often do you receive a good psychiatric report? *CMA Journal, 127,* 697–698.

Silva, J. A., Weinstock, R., & Leony G. B. (2003). Forensic psychiatric report writing. In R. Rosner (Ed.), *Principles and practice of forensic psychiatry* (2nd ed., chapter 4, pp. 31–36). London: Arnold.

Wettstein, R. (2004). The forensic examination and report. In R. I. Simon & L. H. Gold (Ed.), *Textbook of forensic psychiatry* (chapter 7, pp. 139–159, esp. 154–158). Washington, DC: American Psychiatric Publishing.

Appendix C

ADJUNCTIVE USE OF TESTS, INVENTORIES, SURVEYS, AND OTHER INSTRUMENTS AND ASSESSMENT TOOLS IN FORENSIC MENTAL HEALTH EVALUATIONS

The use of various tests, inventories, surveys, and other such instruments and investigations in forensic mental health evaluations can be useful to the examiner in several ways, as they are recommended and have been used in the evaluation reports discussed in this book. As such, the use of tests and assessment tools may be considered as adjuncts or supplements to a clinically directed interview/examination conducted by the forensic mental health professional.

Table C.1 lists several applications of testing in forensic evaluations.

Adjunctive tests and investigations from a clinical perspective consist of a wide variety of techniques, medical methods and methodologies, scientific technology, and instruments. Table C.2 gives an overview of those various methodologies and techniques, presented in four broad categories.

Focusing on the last category of tests and assessment tools—the "pencil and paper" tests—the testing literature includes literally thousands of tests in many areas of application (e.g., psychological, vocational, educational, neurological, neuropsychological, and many others) that have been developed over the years. A review of even a small representative sample of the wide range of available tests is clearly beyond the scope of this appendix and this book.

However, for present purposes, "pencil and paper" tests, inventories, surveys, and other instruments may be categorized in several ways. These are: (a) standardized versus nonstandardized tests; (b) self-report tests versus tests

C.1 Applications of Tests, Inventories, Surveys, and Other Instruments in Forensic Mental Health Evaluations

- Obtain additional historical information beyond clinical interview and examination (surveys)
- Standardized data and profiles to compare subjects with others in population (standardized tests)
- For follow-up purposes and to monitor changes over time (all testing)
- Assess distortion and malingering in subjects (MMPI-2 especially)

C.2   Methods and Techniques of Clinical Testing

- Body fluid/laboratory testing (blood, urine, saliva, sweat, semen)
- Electrodiagnostic testing (EKG, EEG, EMG, BEAM, nerve conductive studies)
- Radiographic and imaging techniques (diagnostic X-rays, CT and MRI scanning, PET and SPECT scanning, and others)
- Psychological/neuropsychological tests, surveys, questionnaires, and other standardized and nonstandardized tests and inventories ("paper and pencil" tests)

administered, scored, and interpreted by psychological technicians, psychologists, and other professionals; and (c) surveys for testing and related data collection versus psychological testing that assesses test and inventory subjects in terms of test constructs based on personality and diagnostic concepts, and constructs as presented and discussed in the current edition of the *Diagnostic and Statistical Manual of Mental Disorders, Fourth Edition, Text Revision,* or *DSM-IV-TR,* © 2000, of the American Psychiatric Association. The tests often administered as a nonstandardized test battery by the first-named author of this book include examples of categories (a) and (c), with referrals when indicated to psychologists for category (b) testing.

Table C.3 lists the individual tests in this battery, indicating what category and type apply to each test.

Brief summaries of each of these tests and inventories follow:

C.3   Nonstandardized Test Battery Used in This Book

- Minnesota Multiphasic Personality Inventory, 2nd edition, or MMPI-2 (standardized)
- Millon Clinical Multiaxial Inventory, 3rd edition, or MCMI-III (standardized)
- Beck Depression Inventory, 2nd edition, or BDI-II (standardized)
- Addiction Assessment Questionnaire (nonstandardized; survey)
- Michigan Alcohol Screening Test, or MAST (standardized; survey)
- Drug Abuse Screening Test, or DAST (standardized; survey)
- Alcohol Use Disorders Identification Test, or AUDIT (standardized; survey)
- Mini-Mental State Examination, or MMSE (standardized; administered by forensic mental health professional)
- Cognitive Capacity Screening Examination, or CCSE (standardized; administered by forensic mental health professional)
- Past Medical History, or PMH (nonstandardized; survey)

1. The MMPI-2 is a 567-item, or 567-question, standardized psychological objective personality assessment inventory used to develop clinical profiles of test subjects in comparison with the general population, or subject of the population (e.g., correctional trusties). This test has scales that identify distortions, exaggerations, and inconsistencies during responses. These distortions, depending on their nature, extent, and pattern, may be interpreted as "feeling good" or "feeling bad." This test may be computer-scored and interpreted or hand-scored and interpreted by psychologists or psychological technicians.

2. The MCMI-III is similar to the MMPI-2, but with fewer true-false test items or questions; 175 items. This inventory is also a standardized psychological objective personality inventory. Unlike the MMPI-2 this test does not assess for feeling. The first-named author of this book, Dr. Greenfield, uses both the MMPI-2 and the MCMI-III as cross-checking devices.

3. The BDI-II is a standardized self-report test for symptoms of depression in which the test-taker is instructed to respond to the test items for the two-week period leading up to and including the day of the test being self-administered.

4. The Addiction Assessment questionnaire is a nonstandardized survey instrument for taking a chemical dependency and treatment (chemical dependency and/or psychiatric) history.

5. The MAST is a standardized self-report instrument intended to yield responses comparing the test-taker's alcohol history with that of others taken with this instrument (i.e., to obtain normative statistical epidemiologic data about the test-taker concerning alcohol use history).

6. The DAST is similar and analogous to the MAST, but focuses on the test-taker's drug use rather than alcohol. It also yields normative statistical epidemiological data about the test-taker's reported drug use testing.

7. The AUDIT is another self-report standardized instrument intended to compare the test-taker's alcohol use history with that of others measured with this instrument. The first-named author of this book, Dr. Greenfield, uses both the MAST and the AUDIT as cross-checks on each other.

8. The MMSE is a standardized cognitive screening instrument—in effect, a simple IQ test—that is used to establish a basic cognitive level of competence (i.e., to proceed with the forensic interview/examination or not) of the test-taker. It also provides normative data that permits the test administrator to rank the test with standardized scores in terms of mild, moderate, and severe cognitive impairment. It is administered to the test-taker by the psychiatrist or psychologist.

9. The CCSE is similar to the MMSE. Both are used by the first-named author as cross-checks on each other.

10. The PMH inventory is a nonstandardized survey instrument either used as a self-report or administered by the psychiatrist or psychologist to supplement the medical history taken by the administrator and to cross-check with information contained in records reviewed and/or provided by the subject.

The adjunctive use of the instruments and assessment tools described in this appendix can be very useful to the forensic mental health professional in conducting evaluations. The literature is replete with discussions of these tools, their scope and functions, the relevant methodologies, how they operate, and other information as presented in Appendix C.

However, in the final analysis, forensic evaluations conducted by mental health professionals addressing the types and scope of issues discussed in this book are clinically based, and rely on clinical methodologies and approaches. While the tools and instruments presented and discussed in this appendix can provide adjunctive or supplementary information to the forensic examiner, they should not and cannot substitute for, or replace, the clinical core of the forensic mental health evaluation, the interview/examination of the subject.

Index